MW00647111

Yoga Sequences Companion

Yoga Sequences Companion

A TREASURE TROVE FOR
STUDENTS AND TEACHERS

VANI DEVI

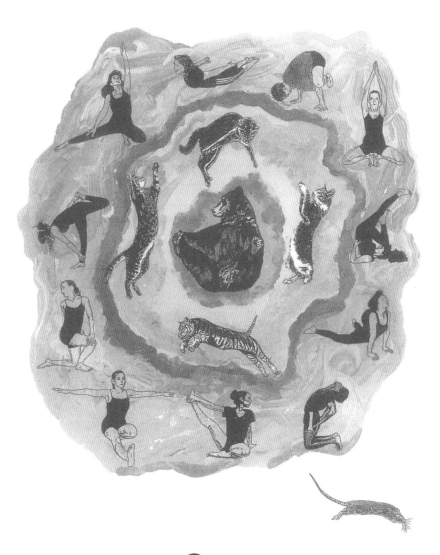

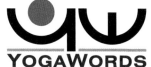

YOGAWORDS

The writer and publisher of this book do not accept responsibility for any accident, injury or problem caused by practising the breath work, meditations or postures in this book. Not all postures and practices are appropriate for all people. It is your responsibility to know your body and its limitations and to choose suitable practices. Please read the 'Cautions and Health Issues' section before commencing your practice and consult a medical practitioner if necessary.

First published in 2011 by Kool Kat Publications

This edition published by YogaWords 2015, reprinted 2017

Text and illustrations © Vani Devi / Kool Kat Publications 2011

All rights reserved

ISBN 978-1-906756-35-2

Vani Devi has asserted her moral right to be identified as the author of this work in accordance with the copyright, designs and patents act of 1988.

A catalogue record for this book is available from the British library.

This book is sold subject to the condition that it shall not, by way of trade and otherwise, be lent, resold, hired out, or otherwise circulated without the publisher's prior consent in any form or binding or cover other than that in which it is published and without a similar condition being imposed on the subsequent purchaser. The author and publisher disclaim, as far as the law allows, any liability arising directly or indirectly from the use, or misuse, of the information contained in this book.

Interior designed and edited by Andy Wood.

Printed and bound in the EU by Hussar Books.

This book has been printed on paper that is sourced and harvested from sustainable forests.

Published by YogaWords
An imprint of Pinter and Martin Ltd
6 Effra Parade
London SW2 1PS

www.pinterandmartin.com

The author can be reached at:
Vani Devi, 1 Dene Way, Newbury, RG14 2JL, UK
www.koolkatpublications.co.uk

Contents

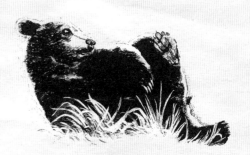

Yoga: Definitions and Quotations

THE WORD yoga is derived from the Sanskrit root *yog*, which means *union* or *contact*. It corresponds to the two English verbs: to *join* or to *unite*. It is sometimes linked to the English word *yoke*. Sanskrit words have a way of accumulating meaning and definitions. If you read any book that is trying to explain about yoga, you are likely to discover different meanings and definitions of the word. Often the writer is giving us their own interpretation of this wonderful tradition.

Here are some interpretations I have come across:
In the *Bhagavad Gita* it says yoga is *balance*. George Feuerstein has called it *discipline*. In a workshop, Kausthub Desikachar said it meant *protection*, *connection* and *meditation*.

Here are some definitions:
From Terri Hector we have: *Yoga is a way of storing Universal energy within the human body.*
From two forgotten sources: *Yoga is a voyage of inner discovery and a way of living creatively in a sacred presence.*
George Feuerstein says: *Yoga is a means of contacting your inner happiness.*
From a *Self Knowledge Journal* handout: *Yoga is an investigation into the ultimate nature of our being.*
From Swami Nishchalananda Saraswati: *Yoga is a process of being open to the vast arena of the unknown, without credulity or naivety.*
From Mohini Chatlani: *Yoga is an internal journey to the magic of becoming light and empowered.*
The most frequently quoted definition comes from the *Yoga Sutras of Patanjali*: *Yoga is a process of uniting the individual soul with the Universal Soul. Yoga is also that state in which the activities of the mind are restrained.*

Here are some quotations which expand and illuminate the above:

From the Victorian poet, Lord Alfred Tennyson: *A kind of waking trance I have had, quite up from boyhood, when I have been all alone. This has often come upon me through repeating my own name to myself silently till, all at once, out of the intensity of the consciousness of individuality, the individuality itself seemed to dissolve and fade away into boundless being; and this is not a confused state, but the clearest of the clearest, surest of the surest, the weirdest of the weirdest, utterly beyond words, where death was almost a laughable impossibility, the loss of personality (if so it were) seemed no extinction, but only true life.*

From Albert Einstein: *Human Beings are part of the whole, called by us 'the universe', a part limited in time and space. One experiences oneself, one's thoughts and feelings as something separate from the rest, which is a kind of optical delusion of consciousness. This delusion is a kind of prison for us, restricting us to our personal desire and the affections of a few persons nearest to us. Our task must be to free ourselves from this prison by widening our circle of compassion to all living creatures and the whole of nature in its beauty. Striving for such an achievement is in itself a part of the liberation and the foundation of inner security.*

From Marques Riviere: *Everybody creates their own Yoga, and if the great rules of Yoga are simple, the practical methods are multiple. It may be said that each individual has their own yoga and exact formula which corresponds to his temperament, to his psychic state ... and his past karma.*

From George Feuerstein: *The emphasis in yoga is always on experimentation and personal verification rather than mere belief.*

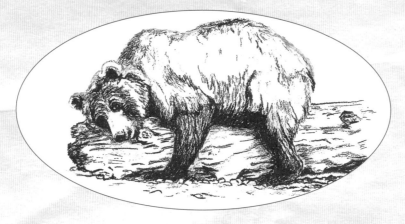

Foot notes
Please refer to the **Glossary** for explanations of Sanskrit and *Bhagavad Gita*.
All quotations by George Feuerstein come from *Living Yoga*. This contains articles from the *Yoga Journal*. 1993, Jeremy P. Tarcher/Putnam. ISBN 0-87477-729-1
Terri Hector is a colleague, and author of *A Breath Behind Time*.
The web site for *Self Knowledge Journal* is www.shantisadan.org
The quotation by Swami Nishchalananda comes from his book *The Edge of Infinity*, Mandala Yoga Ashram, ISBN 0-9544662-1-7.
The quotation by Mohini Chatlani comes from her book *Yoga Flows*, ISBN 1-903-258-33-2
This translation of the *Patanjali Sutra (Samadhi Pada, Sutra 1)* comes from the *Sivananda Advanced Yoga Teacher Manual*.
The quotation by Marques Riviere comes from his book *Tantrik Yoga*, 1970, Rider and Co. and Samuel Weiser. ISBN 877728-006-1

The Glossary

Advaita Vedanta. The **creator** and the **created** are considered one and the same. Matter is energy vibrating at different frequencies. This echoes Einstein's equation, $E=MC^2$, meaning **energy = matter**. The different dimensions and spiritual landscapes are energy functioning in different ways. In some philosophies and religions the **creator** and the **created** are two separate entities.

Ashram. Usually a secluded residence of a spiritual community with teachers, and often based around a particular Guru.

Bhagavad Gita. This is a dialogue between Lord Krishna and Arjuna, from about 2,000 BC. It was transmitted orally for many generations and finally narrated by Vyasa in about 550 BC.

Hatha Yoga. This is one of the four paths of yoga as described by Lord Krishna in the Bhagavad Gita (about 400 BC), see page **9**. Hatha Yoga develops the full potential of the body and mind through systematic practices. These include Asanas (posture work to keep the body fit and connected to the brain), Pranayama (see below) to utilize the vast energy potential in a human being, and meditation to utilize the full potential of the mind.

Hatha Yoga Pradipika. This is a classic Sanskrit manual, written by Swami Svatmarama in about the 15th century AD. It is derived from old Sanskrit texts and his own yogic experiences. It advises the aspiring yogi on how to develop an intense spiritual practice.

Heart Centre. The area associated with love and compassion in the middle of the chest. For more detail see page **4**.

Mantra. This is a verbal vibration, or resonance, that has a beneficial effect on the body and mind. It can be spoken, sung or thought. It can be one or more syllables, a phrase, a sentence, or many sentences. The Hail Mary in the Roman Catholic Church is a long mantra, but there are longer ones in the Jewish canticles. A mantra is repeated many times and used as a point of concentration to steady the mind. People can make up their own mantras, and sometimes a particular word takes over a person's mind and it appears that a mantra has been given to them. For comments on the traditional approach to mantras, see page **159**.

Maya. This is the rope that binds man to the illusory world. It is the power which makes form appear as reality.

Pranayama. Prana means **life force** and **ayama** means **control**, or **mastering**.
It involves many different methods of breathing. When these are combined with other techniques, such as the **Bandhas** as described on page **148,** our energy potential can be developed.

Pratyahara. Withdrawing the five senses away from the outside world and directing them inwards. For more detail, see page **153**.

Samskaras. Deep mental impressions produced by past experiences. They can be dormant impressions from our past lives.

Sanskrit. This was the language of the ancient civilization which developed on the banks of the Indus River in what is now Pakistan. We find the earliest evidence of yoga here.

Throat Centre. This is the Vishuddha Chakra in the throat. It acts as a bridge between the higher and lower intelligence in the body. What is felt there will be a reflection of the relationships between the abdomen, heart and brain in the head.

Information about the illustrations

People often ask me if my illustrations are drawings or photographs. The answer is that they are both. I take photos of my pupils or colleagues and photocopy them. I trace the outline of the bodies and then stick on the heads from the photocopies, and complete the drawings.

Most of the animal illustrations are taken from two websites: www.istockphoto.com, www.stillpictures.co.uk, and from Google free images. The others come from various sources. I have received permission from nearly all relevant parties. In a few cases I have not been able to trace the publisher or photographer. A special mention is due to Newbury-based bear photographer Andrew Gutteridge. His photographs inspired the bear illustrations on the previous and contents pages, and pages **4** and **145**.

Since illustrating my first Yoga Sequence book in 2003, my technique for producing the illustrations has evolved. In some sequences, for example in the **Gate Sequence** and **Divers Posture Sequence**, you can see both, some of the earlier drawings and the clearer more recent ones.

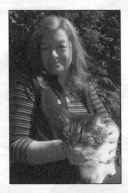

May your yoga bring you joy and contentment.

Love and Light from

Vani Devi

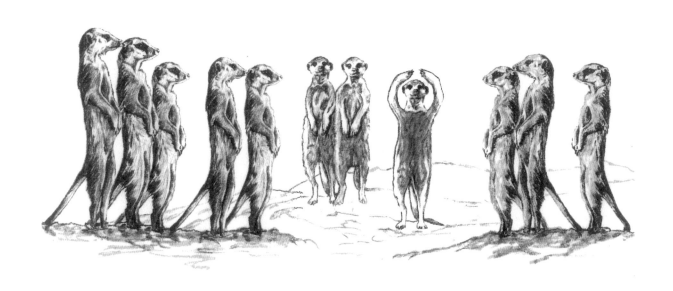

Meerkat Yoga Class

Preface

Yoga Sequences Companion is a compilation of my last three yoga books and additional sequences. I produced the last two books myself at home. This was time-consuming and impractical. I produced *Yoga Expanded and Simplified* without help from anybody and I was never happy with the presentation. As new sequences accumulated, the idea of a manufactured compilation, extending to electronic books (e-books), became more attractive.

To summon the help needed, I placed an advertisement in the local paper; 'Help needed from somebody with experience in publishing'. Andy Wood was one of four people to offer their assistance and this book is the result of our combined efforts.

The style of the book

I teach children the guitar in schools and support adults with special needs in care homes, both part time. I try to appeal to these groups of clientele when I write my books. Yoga has the potential to help everybody. I try to keep the language as simple as possible. At times it is almost colloquial. Although I love the Sanskrit words, I have kept them to a minimum.

Readers tell me they like the animal pictures. They offer light relief and also celebrate nature and the wonders of Creation. Yogi Bhajan, who founded the Kundalini Yoga movement says:

If you can't see God in all, you can't see God at all.

All short quotations are in bold italics (as above). This is to avoid an avalanche of inverted commas. Punctuation is kept to a minimum.

Acknowledgements

The inspirational people and teachers who have helped me with my books are too numerous to mention. I extend my gratitude to them all, especially my pupils. However, Bob Camp and Malcolm Bray deserve a special mention as they have contributed their own sequences. Bob is still teaching yoga in Norwich in his eighties. Malcolm teaches in the Newbury area. Also, editor and designer Andy Wood has been a tower of strength; and proofreader Rachel Tapping, a blessing. I thank them both for their expertise and patience.

My background information

I studied the guitar and singing at the Guildhall School of Music in the 1960s. Kate Oppel is my married name. In my early forties I had a consultation with a Harley Street speech therapist about a problem that developed at the age of ten. The therapist advised me, 'I can't do anything for you but I suggest you take up yoga'. About two years later I finally made it to a local class and yoga has subsequently become an essential part of my life.

I took the Sivananda Yoga Teachers Training Course in the Bahamas in 1998. I was given my spiritual name there. Vani Devi means Goddess of Speech and Song. I started teaching straight away in local village halls and Pinnacle (now Nuffield Health) leisure centre. In 2001 I started teaching at Resource in Reading. This is a drop-in centre supporting people whose lives have been disrupted by mental health problems. I am still teaching at these establishments. In 2001 I took the Sivananda Advanced Course in Canada. This was followed by the Sadana Intensive in the Himalayas in 2004, and again in France in 2005. This course involves studying the *Hatha Yoga Pradipika* and going deeper into the practice of *Pranayama* (exploring the potential of the breath). I have also taught young offenders in Reading Prison and patients in a psychiatric hospital in Reading.

I am very fortunate to be living in an area which is overflowing with yogic activity. I have had the opportunity to explore different styles of posture work, ranging from Dru to Iyengar. In Oxford there is a very active Ashtanga Yoga group and the Inner Book Shop, where I have found some gems in the second-hand book section. Three British Wheel of Yoga Congresses and weekends at the Pastoral Centre in Hatfield have also been catalytic.

As I teach open, mixed ability classes, it has been necessary to develop different ways of practising the postures. Also, as yoga teaching is usually taught in England and other countries in weekly classes or in terms, the class routine becomes part of our pupils lives. I have met some yoga teachers who have been teaching the same pupils for 25 and 40 years on this basis. Although repetition is an essential part of yoga practice, innovation is necessary to keep the lessons interesting and develop potential.

Other books self-published by the Author
Blues Guitar, Play it Your Way. Kate Oppel, 1994.   ISBN 0-9524781-02
Yoga Sequences. Vani Devi, 2003.   ISBN 0-9524781-0
Yoga Sequences. Book 2, 2007.   ISBN 0-9524781-8-8
Yoga Expanded and Simplified. 2009.   ISBN 978-0-9524781-4-0

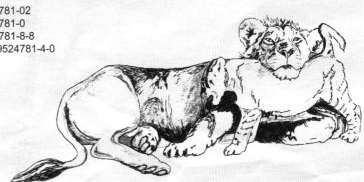

Foreword

IN THIS, her fourth yoga book, Vani Devi has brought together new yoga sequences and material from her earlier works, in a format and presentation that makes it easier to use. She draws on many years of yoga teaching, with a wide variety of students and their specific conditions and needs. This includes young men imprisoned in Reading Young Offenders Institution, to people with mental health issues.

As I practise and follow her clear and uplifting illustrations, I feel more connected to the natural world. Nothing is lost or watered down by this approach. On the contrary, if you are feeling serious, heavy and overly analytical, the images and simplicity allow the mind to relax and feel light. This can lead to a deeper experience of yoga.

While some of the postures are more challenging, the presentation encourages modification, self-respect and breath awareness. These are principles which yoga teachers frequently struggle to have their students embrace. Vani Devi is to be commended for communicating these principles so well. I'm sure you will enjoy using and sharing this book with others as much as she has clearly enjoyed putting it together.

Sam Settle
Director of the Prison Phoenix Trust

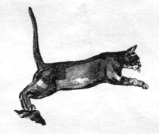

The Heart Centre

The Heart Centre is the Anahata Chakra. Chakra means wheel of energy. It is placed on the same level as the heart but in the centre of the body. This aligns it with the spine and the other energy centres.

In pre-scientific ages the heart was considered to be the symbol of eternity and the true seat of the intellect. It is the place where we know and feel. Belief systems are created in the verbal centres in the left side of the brain[1].

Ongoing research can help us to have a better understanding of the Heart Centre. This following information comes from *Living in the Heart*, by Drunvalo Melchizedek[2]:

Doctors have wondered how the heart of a baby, developing in the womb, begins to beat before the brain is formed. A research group, the Institute of HeartMath, connected to Stanford University in California, discovered the heart has its own brain. It is a very small brain with about 40,000 brain cells, but it is obviously all that the heart needs.

They also proved ... **that the human heart generates the largest and most powerful energy field of any organ in the body, including the brain within the skull ... This electromagnetic field is about 8 - 9 feet in diameter, with its axis centred in the heart ... Heart surgeons have found that there is a tiny space within the heart that must never be touched for any reason or the person will immediately die.**

The quotation below is from *Chandogya Upanishad, 8.1.2 - 3*. I have spaced the lines in a particular way to point the meaning:

If someone says to you,
'In the fortified city of the imperishable, our body,
there is a lotus and in this lotus a tiny space:
What does it contain that one should desire to know it?'

You must reply:
'As vast as this space without, is the tiny space within the heart:
Heaven and earth are found in it,
Fire and air, sun and moon,
Lightning and the constellations,
Whatever belongs to you here below and all that doesn't,
All this is gathered in the tiny space within the heart'.

Bears Care

1. *Statistics vary. These statistics come from Wikipedia, the free encyclopedia. About five per cent of right-handed men and ten per cent of right-handed women have their language and speech centres in the right side of the brain. In left-handed people, right hemisphere language dominance is found in about 18.8 per cent and 19.8 per cent have bilateral language functions.*
2. Living in the Heart *by Drunvalo Melchizedek, Technology Publishing, 2003. ISBN 1-891824-43-0*

The Yoga Sequence

A YOGA sequence is made up of **Asana**[1] and **Vinyasa**. An asana is a physical posture that begins with effort and is held in a state of balance and concentration. The asana is found in other traditions, e.g. in ancient Shamanism[2], to induce ecstatic states or out-of-body experiences, and within the wrestling tradition of India.

In yoga the body is the instrument through which spiritual aims are achieved[3]. The sustained effort and concentration of the asana leads to the higher yogic goals.

Legends speak of many thousands of asanas but only a few have been illustrated or described anywhere before the last century. The asana tradition can be described as an oral one (transmitted and preserved by the spoken word). Within any oral tradition we find much variation, as individuals and groups select and add and detract from communicated information. This functions at a conscious and unconscious level.

Vinyasas are postures that link the asanas together. In this book most of the recognised asanas are named, but for the sake of simplicity I have called them both postures. There are many variations in the names of asanas.

When you do the sequence once with the right foot leading and repeat it with the left foot leading it is called **One Round**.

Of all the sequences in this book, I am only aware that the **Sun Salutations**, **Hero Sequence** and the **Five Tibetan Rites** are traditional, i.e. have been handed down through successive generations. When material is transmitted orally it is difficult to trace its history.

Some of the sequences, e.g. the **Sitting Stretch Sequence** and **Abdominal Workout**, may appear to be no more than fitness routines. It is when the philosophy and practices of yoga are applied that they become vehicles of spiritual development.

A further extension of the yoga sequence is found in Kripalu Yoga[4]. Some yogis, throughout the ages, have found that their body suddenly starts to move automatically, as if it had a mind of its own. It just flows from one posture to another. Swami Sivananda says[5], *When you involuntarily perform different Asanas and poses without the least pain or fatigue, know you that the Kundalini[6] has become active.*

Krishnamacharya (1888-1989) said; *It is not for the individual to adapt her/himself to yoga, rather for yoga to adapt itself to the individual.* He taught yoga at the Mysore Palace in southern India. Three of his disciples went on to develop very different schools of posture work. They are P. Jois (Astanga Vinyasa Yoga), his son T.K.V. Desikachar (Vini Yoga), and B.K.S. Iyengar (Iyengar Yoga). Against the vast yogic background, these differences are insignificant. Iyengar himself said; *In yoga ... many may take one path as a key in order to experience self-realization, while others take another path, but I say that there is absolutely no difference between the various practices of yoga.*

A manuscript from the Mysore Palace (dated between 1811 and 1868), contains details and illustrations of 121 asanas. The asanas were practised in the gymnasium and some of them make use of the ropes. One uses two ropes to ascend and the participant has a weight dangling from his mouth. Such is the flexibility of the asana.

You choose the posture work and yogic path that suits your needs. Similarly with the sequences, adapt them to your individual needs.

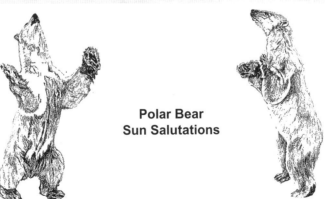

**Polar Bear
Sun Salutations**

1. *The first A of Asana has an accent and is pronounced 'arsana'. The accent is sometimes missed out. Asana means 'to sit'.*
2. *Spiritual healers.*
3. *In this respect a portion of yoga practice comes from the Tantric tradition. This is an ancient tradition that developed simultaneously, quite independently, in various parts of the world. George Feuerstein says; **The tradition of Tantrism has hailed the body as a most valuable instrument for realizing the Divine, or Reality.** This is a very misunderstood tradition. It is often associated with sexual experimentation but one branch of the tradition advises celibacy, The advanced pranayama teachings of the **Hatha Yoga Pradipika** (c. 1400CE) can be described as Tantric.*
4. *Yogi Amrit Desai created Kripalu Yoga in 1970 after experiencing involuntary movements.*
5. *This is from Kundalini Yoga by Swami Sivananda. ISBN 81-7052-052-5*
6. *A particular type of spiritual energy that can awaken in the body.*

Breathing

THE BREATH is very important in yogic thinking. When we inhale we not only take in oxygen, we take in Prana. This is the Life Force or Cosmic Energy, and breathing is our link to the cosmos. Different cultures and religions have their own terminology for the Life Force; for example, it is the **Holy Spirit** in Christianity and **Chi** or **Qui** in China.

When we inhale, we can think of building up this store of energy in the abdomen. It is psychologically healthy to be aware of this grounding, calming and strengthening force in the abdomen. Traditionally, the yogic inhalation has been taken with a relaxed abdomen. When you inhale, your whole trunk from the top of the thighs to half way up the neck should move. Scientists have picked up minute movements in the bones of the skull during the breathing process. As the diaphragm flattens and extends, everything around the waist should move. The relaxed abdomen rises and the whole of the back, including below the waist, should expand. It is possible to breathe without using the diaphragm at all. In yogic breathing we take the air down to the bottom of the lungs and use full lung capacity unless there is a particular reason for changing.

Most people breathe between fifteen and twenty times a minute. The breath is closely linked with mental activity. When we are agitated, we breathe quickly. When we listen acutely, we stop breathing. When we slow down our breathing, we become calm.

Experimenting with breath and emotions

To experience this connection, experiment with feeling different emotions. Observe the speed of your breathing and which parts of the body are moving. Here are some suggestions:

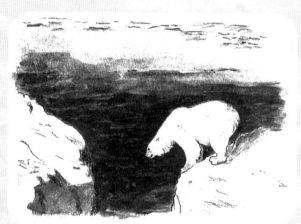

Imagine you are relaxing in a hot bath.

Feel very angry.

You are warm and cosy in bed and about to fall asleep.

Feel very frightened.

Imagine you are stroking an animal you love very much.

Imagine you are an actor or musician about to perform a demanding part.

Feel very happy.

Feel very sad.

Imagine you are about to meet somebody who is important to you. You haven't seen them for a long time and you are both excited and apprehensive.

Our exhalations should be twice as long as our inhalations in everyday life. Practising yoga makes you aware of your breathing and the potential expansion of the rib cage.

How to Breathe in the Sequences

Some of the sequences have obvious breathing patterns, others are more obscure. Usually you inhale as you extend and exhale as you contract. Some teachers like to inhale into a backward bend, others prefer to exhale. Most of the breathing indications are only my suggestions. You may find them pedantic and prefer to forget about them while you learn the sequences. Sometimes just be an observer and watch to see how your breath responds to different postures.

In some of the sequences, it is suggested that you hold the postures. While you do this you can breathe in different ways. You can either breathe as your body dictates or you can consciously make your breathing deeper and slower. It is usual to take between three and eight breaths as you hold a posture but you can take more if you want to. Also, where I have put **Repeat three times**, you can make more repetitions if it feels right.

Changing attitudes towards the Breath

Since writing my first book of sequences, my attitude towards breathing has been influenced by several people.

First, I read an article in a *Yoga and Health* magazine by Bill Heilbronn. It was called 'New thoughts on Kumbhaka[1] in the light of Buteyko'. It states there should be approximately six per cent carbon dioxide in the bloodstream. Lower levels make the blood alkaline (salty), whereas in good health it should veer towards the acidic. Higher levels would cause asphyxiation (suffocation), but lower levels cause the symptoms that are recognised as asthma. This completely changed my attitude towards breathing as I had always thought it best to be highly oxygenated[2].

Since reading the article I have made greater use of the pauses after inhalation and exhalation, especially after exhalation. Buteyko says a healthy person should be able to pause for 40 seconds at the end of a complete exhalation. I was surprised to find that many of my pupils could do this. He says if you can't manage 10 seconds you are likely to have a serious breathing condition.

Then I studied with Sunil Kumar for one week in Varanasi. He had a broad-minded attitude towards breathing (see **Varanasi Sun Salutations**).

I attended a workshop given by osteopath, Peter Blackaby. He explained that you get a better curvature of the spine if you exhale on a backward bend. I had accepted the traditional way of inhaling into **Cat** and **Cobra** and hadn't questioned it, but the curvature of the spine does seem better if you reverse the breathing.

Also my attitude towards abdominal breathing has clarified. Traditionally, the yogic inhalation has been taken with a relaxed abdomen; i.e. the abdomen expands on the inhalation and flattens on the exhalation. This is how animals and babies breathe when they are relaxed. When they are active or agitated, the activity can move higher up into the lungs.

After about 1920 some teachers started to disagree with this approach and suggested a slight contraction of the abdominal muscles on the inhalation. This was influenced by an Indian research institute called Kaivalyadhana. They stated that ... *In the laboratory evidence we have collected ... the controlled abdomen allows at the time more oxygen to be inhaled than the protracted[3] abdomen. So far as the culture of nerves is concerned, controlled abdominal muscles have a decided advantage over protracted abdominal muscles.*

However, those who practise activities that involve taking in large amounts of air on the inhalation, do not restrict the abdomen. As a student of singing at the Guildhall School of Music in the 1960s, I was taught to expand around the waist on the inhalation. The abdominal muscles engage automatically on the exhalation to support the outgoing breath. Consciously manipulating the abdomen takes the enjoyment out of singing.

Also, I had the good fortune to come across a copy of a magazine called *The Week* in my dentist's waiting room. It contained an article about Tanya Streeter who holds the record for deep sea diving. She can hold her breath for six minutes and 17 seconds. She says that when she gets ready to dive, she breathes in so much air that her stomach swells until it looks like she is six months pregnant.

In Pilates, a slight contraction of the abdomen is recommended on the inhalation. This is understandable as Pilates was created with the ballet dancer in mind. An expanded abdomen would spoil the body line for dancing. Also the abdominal muscles support the spine during movement. I went to one yoga class where the teacher taught Pilates breathing and decided it was definitely not for me, but yoga can accommodate differences of opinion.

However, awareness that it is not the traditional yogic method of breathing and that it is a recent mutation is necessary. 'The proof of the pudding is in the eating'. Most people need to breathe with a relaxed abdomen for psychological wellbeing.

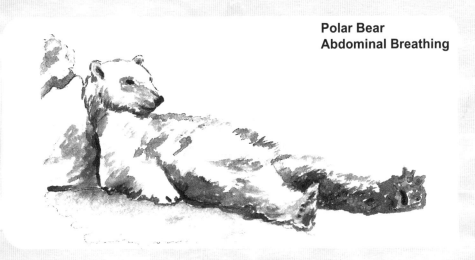

**Polar Bear
Abdominal Breathing**

1. *Kumbhaka is the pause after inhalation and exhalation. For more information about Buteyko go to:* **www. buteykovideo.com**

2. *In more detail: Bill Heilbronn points out in his article;*
There is a popular misunderstanding of carbon dioxide in the respiratory process. It is thought by many that carbon dioxide is only a waste gas caused by the 'burning' of the blood sugar by the oxygen in the blood to fuel the requirements of the muscles, and that together with the water vapour also produced, it must be eliminated as thoroughly as possible.
In fact, this is not the whole story. Carbon dioxide is actually essential. Paradoxically, when carbon dioxide levels in the blood are lowered, the chemical bond between the oxygen and haemoglobin increases. Because the haemoglobin in the red blood cells will not let go of its oxygen, this makes it harder for the cells of the brain, heart and kidneys etc to get the oxygen they need ...

3. *Protracted means drawn out, drawing a part forwards and away from the body.*

Cautions and Health Issues

PEOPLE HURT themselves putting out garbage, turning over in bed, and bending down to pick something up. It is obvious that care must be taken when practising yoga postures. As physical activities go, yoga has a good track record, although one hears of the occasional trapped nerve or accident. Dancers are much more likely to hurt themselves, and athletes and football players have a shorter than average life expectancy.

Most of the feedback I have received about my yoga books has been from yoga teachers. A few people told me they practised from them at home and didn't attend a class. These are the ones who will need extra guidance and I am writing here with them in mind.

I prefer to distinguish between the fit and unfit, the well-coordinated and the uncoordinated, rather than the beginner and non-beginner. Some people do demanding postures with complete composure and confidence in their first yoga class. Some are used to listening to their bodies: others have lost touch with their bodies and need to develop this skill. Patience is also needed. It is important not to try too hard. Always keep within your comfort zone.

Wait until your body has warmed up before practising demanding stretches and twists. Start with some spinal rocks and a gentle sequence like the **Golden Seed** (*see page 134*). You are less likely to hurt yourself if you coordinate your breath with your posture work. Always connect to the breath. Stop if there is any discomfort. Don't hold the postures for too long at first. Move slowly and carefully from one posture to another.

Here are some recognized precautions

If you have a particular physical problem, consult a medical practitioner. Advice varies; if in doubt, seek a second opinion.

If you have **high blood pressure** it is advisable not to lower the head below the hips, unless you are used to doing this with no ill effects. Care is also needed with inverted postures, e.g. the **Head Stand** and **Shoulder Stand**. Taking the hips above the head may not be advisable, although some people with high blood pressure are quite comfortable in inverted postures.

Pregnant women should lie on their left-hand side during relaxation. Also they should not put pressure on the abdomen by lying face downwards.

If you have **heart problems** or are **pregnant**, don't hold your breath for more than about ten seconds.

Avoid inverted postures (see above) if you suffer from **glaucoma, detached retina**, **neck problems**, or have an **ear infection**. This also applies if you have had **eye surgery**. Some **pregnant** women are fine doing them: others may faint or have difficulty, so proceed with great caution.

Neck and **back** problems vary greatly. Find out which postures help your condition and avoid those that don't. Your medical practitioner should be able to advise you if necessary.

If you have taken **pain killers**, take care not to over-stretch during posture work as signals to the brain will be suppressed.

If you have had a **hip replacement**, avoid movements like the **Swinging Gate** in the **Gate Sequence**. Follow the advice of your medical practitioner.

Things you need to know

Ujjayi breathing is mentioned throughout the book. Please read **Throat and Nose Breathing** on page 154, before starting the sequences. Also you will need to read The **Sympathetic and Parasympathetic Nervous Systems** on page 155, before you start the **Lion's Roar Sequence**. Knowledge of these nervous systems will benefit your meditation and general well-being. It is essential reading.

Venus Lock is also mentioned throughout the book. The fingers are interlocked and the palms usually pushed away.

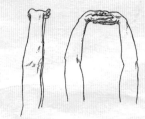

Venus Lock

A few thoughts to dwell on before you start your posture work

During the day we get used to repeating the same movements over and over again. Sometimes a group of muscles will not be used for a long time and their pathway to the brain can almost go to sleep. Just waking up these pathways and connecting your body to the brain again is beneficial on all levels. I constantly remind unfit new pupils that their postures don't have to be perfect. It is sufficient at first to use muscles that have not been used for some time. It is beneficial to move the body in lots of different ways. When energy blockages are released and energy flows more freely in the body, the benefits will be felt.

Yoga is an education in breathing. Many people breathe in an unhealthy way. Yoga can correct this. You are never too old to take up yoga. I took my Yoga Teachers Training course at the age of 52. I wasn't particularly flexible. By the time I reached my 60s, I was much more flexible and I had more energy.

Here are a few thoughts from yoga teacher Sylvia Smith. *My own 'mantras' in class are the words 'effortless effort' and 'no two bodies are the same'. Movement is Life. The medical experts agree that to keep moving, even though it might be slightly uncomfortable at times, is to keep the energy circulating.*

LORD KRISHNA, who lived about 2000BC, spoke about these four paths. His teachings were transmitted orally for many generations and finally narrated in the *Bhagavad Gita* (c.600-500BC).

Karma Yoga, the Yoga of Action. This is selfless service towards our fellow human beings, the Planet Earth and the Higher Consciousness with no thought of personal reward. Deeds, not words are important. The good and bad usage of words corresponds to deeds.

Bhakti Yoga, the Yoga of Devotion. This is an emotional longing for involvement with the cosmos and Higher Consciousness. Words are not used to justify the emotion but to express it in singing and chanting, ceremony, ritual, and story-telling.

Raja Yoga, the Yoga of Meditation. This is mind control with a goal to achieving higher states of consciousness. The asanas and contents of this book belong to this path. The body is controlled as a prelude to controlling the mind. Particular attention is paid to the movement of prana (life force) in the body. This is **Hatha Yoga**. The asana is one of several techniques used for controlling the life force in Hatha Yoga. In Raja Yoga words become superfluous; 'I don't think, therefore I am'.

Jnana Yoga, the Yoga of Knowledge. It uses the intellect to ask questions, read, reflect and analyse. It transcends the unreal and negates bondage to the material world. It is dependent on words until the mind transcends the intellect.

All paths lead to the union of the individual self with the universal self. You are advised to follow the path that suits your personality, but to practise all the other paths to some degree. The usage of words is my own suggestion, to simplify the understanding.

As we hold the postures in a state of bodily concentration and words become superfluous, we may, without realizing it, experience this union, if only for a split second. The same applies during the usual final relaxation in a yoga class, and when we meditate in the postures.

The Eight Limbs of Raja Yoga

Patanjali compiled and explained the most important elements of yogic theory and practice. 2,000 years ago there were many different schools of yoga and some clarification was necessary. This compilation of yoga sutras represents a climax in thousands of years of yogic development.

It is the practical content of the ***Patanjali Sutras*** that have received the most recognition. This includes *The Eight Limbs of Raja Yoga*. Some consider them to be 'the backbone' of yoga.

Limbs, steps or stages of Raja Yoga

1. **Yama**, social conduct. 2. **Niyama**, personal conduct. 3. **Asanas**, postures.
4. **Pranayama**, control of prana, life-force, cosmic energy through breathing. 5. **Pratyahara**, withdrawal of the senses.
6. **Dharana**, concentration. 7. **Dhyana**, meditation. 8. **Samadhi**, the bliss or super-conscious state.

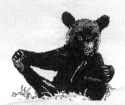

Meditating in the postures

To take your practice to a higher level you can meditate in the postures. You can keep your eyes closed and take a trip **inwards**. This is **withdrawing the senses** (**Pratyahara** in Sanskrit) and the fifth step (limb) in Patanjali's *Eight Steps of Raja Yoga*. You can temporarily disconnect from Planet Earth and when you return you will see things from a different perspective.

At a wonderful weekend at the Mandala Ashram in South Wales, we meditated in the postures using the mantra **So Hum**. This is sometimes translated to mean **I am that I am** but you may prefer to forget this and just concentrate on the vibrations. **Inhale** as you think **So** and **exhale** as you think **Hum**. Say or sing the mantra aloud a few times and then close your eyes and internalize the vibrations. Now add this to your posture work.

You will find that your breathing gets slower and slower, deeper and deeper, and noisier and noisier. As you progress you extend the pauses between the inhalation and exhalation, and vice versa. You can also be aware of the colours you see when your eyes are closed.

In some sequences, e.g. **Salutations to the Sun** and **Moon**, you should keep to the breathing pattern. All the repeated postures, where I have put ***Repeat three times***, can be used. In sequences like the **Canoe** and **Sitting Side Stretch** I hold some of the postures and coordinate the others with the breath. **The Four Directions** and the **Cat Sequence** work well.

Most people achieve a deep state of relaxation and peace during this practice.

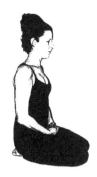

1. Rest your hands in **Zen** position, with the palms facing upwards and the right hand on top, as illustrated.

The Compassionate Breath

Introduction

Sit in any comfortable position. If you are sitting on the floor you can use blocks or cushions to raise the hips a little.

Try to make each exhalation twice as long as the inhalation (*see page 6*).

You can keep to the basic movements and not include all my emotional suggestions or pauses. For example, you can do a simplified version before the **Gaia Sequence** using the **Haaa Breath** (*see pages 14-15*).

A teacher teaching it to a class will, very probably, interpret it in their own way and adjust it to suit their pupils.

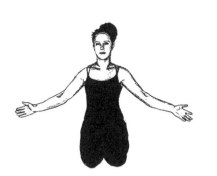
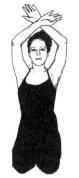

2. As you **INHALE** bring the hands out to the side and above your head. Cross the wrists over with the right hand in front and the palms facing forwards. *Repeat five times.*

Change the hands over so that the left hand is on top in **Zen** position and the left wrist in front above the head. *Repeat five times.*

This requires coordination and concentration. It steadies the mind and prepares it for the rest of the sequence.

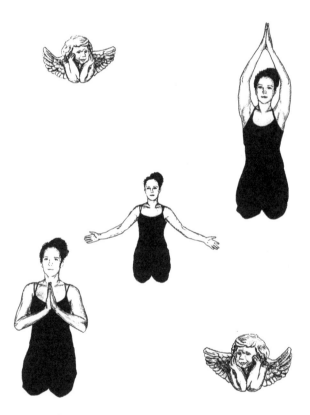

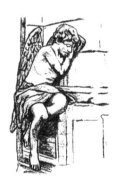

7. Slowly bring your hands back to the **Heart Centre** and place them in **Prayer** position. When you are ready, **INHALE** the hands up above your head.

EXHALE them out to the sides and return them to the **Heart Centre**. *Repeat three times.*

*1. I took a course with Dr Uma Krishnamurti at the Sivananda City Ashram in London in August 2010. She comes from a long line of yogis and was brought up surrounded by yoga. She became a psychiatrist in India and has much experience working with children and adults. She advised us to **linger in the good moments**. During the five days we spent with her, I observed her following her own advice with great skill, prolonging and relishing all the good moments.*

*2. This is written with the beautiful Prayer by St Francis of Assisi, **Make me an Instrument of Your Peace**, in mind.*

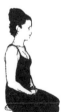

8. Return the hands to **Zen** position, as in **1**, and breathe slowly and gently.

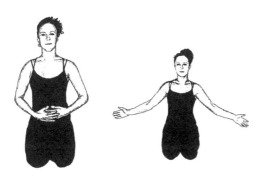

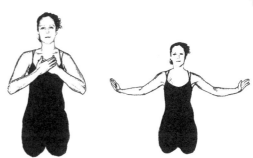

3. Place both hands on the abdomen with one hand on top of the other. As you **INHALE** float your hands out to the sides.

As you **EXHALE** bring them back and place the other hand on top. Repeat five times.

When you **INHALE** open your mind to the vast abundance of creation and to the infinite possibilities it can bestow.

When you **EXHALE** them back, feel contentment, security and peace filling the abdomen and replenishing your energy and emotional strength.

When you have finished, pause for a few breaths to allow yourself to linger with these positive feelings[1]. Gently smile into the abdomen.

4. Move your hands up to the **Heart Centre.** Repeat as in **3**, **INHALING** the hands out and **EXHALING** them back, placing a different hand on top each time. ***Repeat five times.***

When you **INHALE** the hands outwards, let all bad feeling dissolve. Allow all negativity and heaviness that has built up in the mind and body to float away.

When you **EXHALE** them back, feel emotional warmth and allow your heart to soften. Invite love, light, kindness and forgiveness into your heart.

Pause and linger in this tranquil moment for a few breaths. Smile down into the **Heart Centre.**

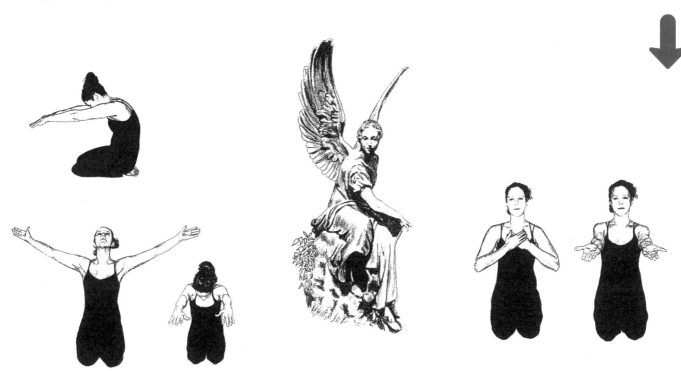

6. Angel Wings: Imagine you are an angel. As you **INHALE** open out your wings and look up to the mysterious and magical 'above and beyond'.

As you **EXHALE** fold your wings forwards. You can slump your back and round your shoulders, stretching them forwards. Turn the palms downwards and push the hands away in front.

Repeat about three times and pause on the last exhalation. Stay for a few breaths with your wings folded and feel as if you are sheltering and cradling under your wings all who need comfort, guidance and protection.

5. Giving and Receiving: Start as in **4**, with the hands on the heart. You receive on the **INHALATION** and give on the **EXHALATION.**

As you **INHALE** with the hands on your heart, allow yourself to receive the goodness, love and abundance of the Universe. Breathe in the wonder of creation.

As you **EXHALE,** stretch out your hands in front with the palms facing upwards. Send peace and love back to the Universe. Let emotional warmth flow from your heart to all who are in need. Offer yourself as an **instrument of peace**[2].

Repeat about three times and pause on the last **EXHALATION.** Stay for a few breaths with the hands stretched out and linger in the moment.

Whole Body Warm-Up Sequence

Body Temperature

THE BODY should be warm before you start stretching and holding postures. During your practice make sure the body temperature doesn't drop. If you are still cold after doing the **Full Body Warm Up**, move on to a few rounds of **Sun Salutations**. Follow this with the **Canoe Sequence**.

During your posture work, energy blockages will be released and pockets of toxins will be dispersed. They will find their way into the lymphatic system and blood stream so that they can be removed from the body. Abdominal breathing also helps this process.

At the end of your posture practice you should relax for about 10-20 minutes. This is usually done lying on your back, palms upwards and with the feet slightly apart in the **Corpse Pose**. This is an important part of your practice. As body temperature is likely to drop when you stop moving, you can cover yourself with a blanket or get into a sleeping bag for this final relaxation.

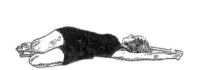

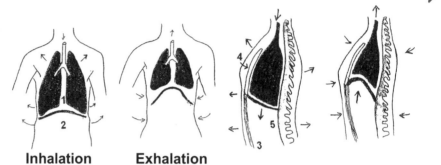

Inhalation   **Exhalation**
1. Lungs **2.** Diaphragm **3.** Abdominal muscles **4.** Rib cage **5.** Spine

13. At the end of your warm up, lie on your back with the knees raised and your hands behind your head in **Venus Lock**. Push away with the palms of the hands. **EXHALE** the knees to the left. Keep the shoulders on the floor and look straight ahead.
Hold the posture and bring your awareness to the breath. The whole of your body, from the top of the thighs to half way up the neck, should move in healthy breathing (scientists have even measured minute movement in the bones of the skull).
Feel the abdomen rising and falling. Locate the diaphragm and become aware of its movement. Bring your awareness to the ribcage and feel the ribs expanding and contracting as you breathe in and out.

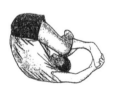

12. Rock backwards and forwards. Try to get your feet to the floor behind you.

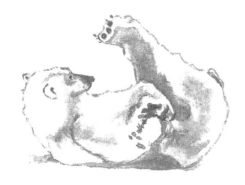

Roly-poly Polar Bear

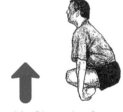

11. Sit at the front of your mat with the legs crossed. Catch hold of your toes with the hands on the outside of the legs. You are going to rock backwards and forwards. Start by bringing your head forward and lifting the hips off the floor to gather momentum.

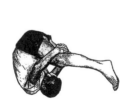

10. Lie on your back and lift the feet towards the ceiling. Straighten the knees and bring the toes towards the head. Catch hold of the thighs or calves and interlock the fingers. Rock backwards and forwards and try to get your feet to the floor behind.
Caution: Avoid **10** and **11** if you have back problems.

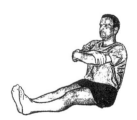

9. Sit up with the legs straight in front. Catch hold of your elbows with your hands. Shuffle forwards, moving one hip at a time, in the **Sitting Walk**. After about 12 shuffles, shuffle back to your starting point. Repeat if you want to.

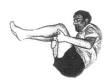

1. Lie on your back. Bring the knees to the chest. Place your hands under the knees and rock backwards and forwards in the **Spinal Rock**.

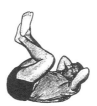

2. Cross the feet over and interlock the fingers behind your head. Bring your head towards the knees and rock backwards and forwards in the **Abdominal Rock**.

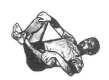

3. Place the hands on the knees and rock from side to side in the **Cradle Rock**.

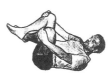

4. With the feet still crossed, circle the knees and pelvis clockwise. You can start off with a small circle and gradually increase it to a large circle. The knees can be closer together for the small circles. *Change direction.*
Now start with a large circle and slowly reduce it. Afterwards, you can place your palms on the floor and rock vigorously backwards and forwards. Try to get your feet to the floor behind.

Introduction
MAKE SURE your back is well cushioned with a thick foam mat. A blanket will not give sufficient protection for the spine. Wear loose, stretchy clothing. An elasticated waistband is essential. Use a non-slip mat if possible and avoid practising straight after a meal.

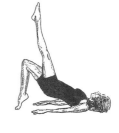

5. Place the left foot over the right knee. Catch hold of your right thigh with both hands and rock backwards and forwards.

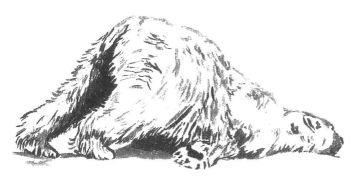

Polar Bear Cooling Down Posture
Polar bears get very hot as they chase after prey across the snow and ice. To lower their body temperature, they press their chest down onto the cold snow.

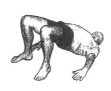
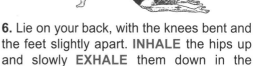

8. Lie on your back. Catch hold of your elbows with your hands. With the knees touching, use your heels to role your body from side to side in the **Full Body Roll**.

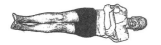

7. Lower the hips and then lift them about 6-inches off the floor. Keeping the knees still and swing the hips from side to side. Press down with the palms in the **Hammock Swing**.
Move the feet further apart and go up on your heels. Swing the hips vigorously from side to side in the **Wide Hammock Swing**.

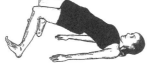

6. Lie on your back, with the knees bent and the feet slightly apart. **INHALE** the hips up and slowly **EXHALE** them down in the **Bridge**. **Repeat three times.**
You can try some variations in the **Bridge**. With the right heel on or off the floor, lift the left leg. Bring your hands behind your head and place the left foot over the right knee. Hold and breathe, lifting the hips as high as you can.
Change sides and repeat.

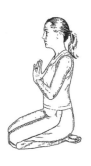

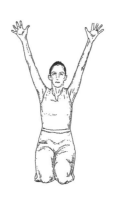

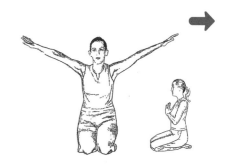

1. Sit in **Thunderbolt** posture, with the buttocks on your heels. If you find this uncomfortable (people who run a lot tend to have difficulty with this pose), find another sitting position. Place the hands in **Prayer** at the **Heart Centre**.

2. INHALE through the nose as you raise your hands above your head.

3. EXHALE with a **Haaaa** breath, through the mouth, as you swing your hands down and out in a circular movement, bringing them back to **1**.
Repeat three times.

Gaia Sequence
Honouring Planet Earth

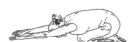

17. Return to **14**.

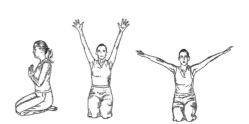

18. When you feel ready, return to **1** and repeat **2** and **3**, three times. Slow down your breathing.
As you INHALE the hands up, concentrate on gathering energy. When you EXHALE the hands down, concentrate on bringing the energy back to the **Heart Centre**.
Return to normal breathing. Close your eyes and breathe into the Heart Centre for a few breaths.

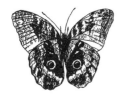

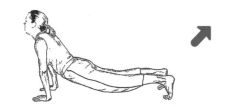

16. INHALE into **Upward Dog**.

15. EXHALE into **Downward Dog**.

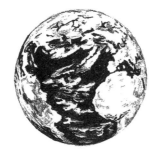

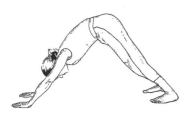

14. Return to **Sphinx** and then EXHALE into **Extended Child's Pose**. Rest for a few breaths, and appreciate the beauty of Planet Earth. **Honour Gaia**.

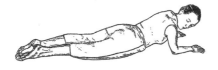

13. EXHALE as you look over your right shoulder.
Repeat three times.

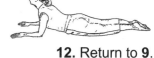

12. Return to **9**.

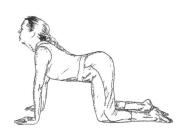 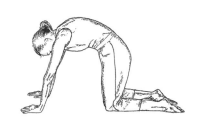 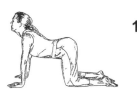

4. INHALE on to your hands and knees into **Upward Cat**.

5. EXHALE into **Downward Cat**. Flatten the abdomen and tuck in the tail bone.
Repeat three times.

6. INHALE again into **Upward Cat**.

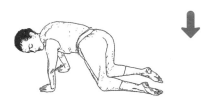

7. EXHALE into **Cat Looks at its Tail**. Move the hips to the left and look round over your left shoulder. Make a **C shape** from the end of your spine and outside of your hips, to the neck and your right ear.
Repeat three times.
Change sides and repeat.

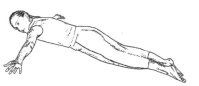

8. Honour Gaia. Lie in a prone posture (face downwards). Stretch your arms out to the side. Look to the left.
Connect to the energy of Planet Earth. Feel thankful for your embodied existence on this beautiful planet and for the range of emotions and experiences it generates[1].

The Haaaa Breath

THE HAAAA breath is not used in yoga as much as it is in Tibetan Healing and Chinese posture work. It involves **inhaling through the nose** and **exhaling through the mouth.**

It can be **voiced**, with a loud Ha, but it is usually **unvoiced**, i.e. whispered and similar to **Ujjayi** breathing.

The vowel sound does not have to be an **Ah**. It can be a neutral sound like **Er.** The **H** consonant at the beginning gives it definition.

Some teachers feel it can be used for emotional release, like a sigh.

In the Gaia Sequence the **Haaaa Breath** can be used most of the time. It adds a feeling of reverence to the sequence. You can use normal breathing when you **Honour Gaia** in **8** and **11**, and also with **Extended Child's Pose** in **14** and **17**.

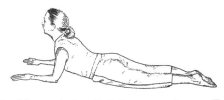

9. Move into **Sphinx posture**. Rest your forearms on the floor. **INHALE** as you lift the head and chest. The abdomen stays on the floor. You can experiment with the positioning of your feet. It is most demanding if the heels and feet touch. Allow the feet to separate if necessary, to ease the lower back.
Place the spine in a **neutral tilt**[2], and slant the hips towards the thighs. Hold for three **Haaaa** breaths.

1. In his consciousness-expanding book The Cosmic Game, *Stanislav Grof explores the relationship between matter and spirit.*
He says ... **The worlds of matter and spirit are coexistent and each has something the other needs ... Spirit has a profound desire to experience what is opposite and contrary to its own nature.**
He talks of **Cosmic Boredom.**
Do spirit entities queue up to be embodied to avoid monotony and to experience the daily phenomena, drama and emotions we consider to be 'part and parcel' of our Earth-bound existence?

2. The curvature of the spine in **Upward Cat** *is called* **Dog tilt.**
The curvature of the spine in **Downward Cat** *is called* **Cat tilt.**
Neutral tilt *is somewhere between the two with the spine like a table top.*

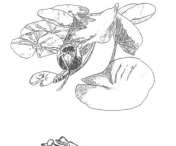
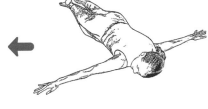
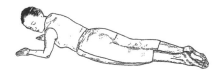

11. Return to **8**. **Honour Gaia** but this time with your head turned to the right.

10. EXHALE as you look over your left shoulder. **INHALE** back to **9**.
Repeat three times.

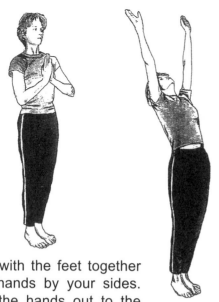

1. Stand with the feet together and the hands by your sides. **INHALE** the hands out to the sides and **EXHALE** them into **Prayer** position.

2. INHALE as you stretch the arms upwards and lean slightly backwards, expanding the rib cage.

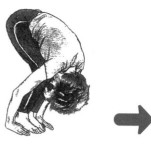

3. EXHALE as you lower the hands to the floor, fingers in line with the toes. Bend your knees and bring your head to your knees.

Salutations to the Sun

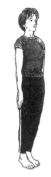

12. EXHALE as you lower your hands to your sides.
Repeat, changing legs on 4 and 9.
This will complete one round. The rounds are usually repeated between five and 40 times.

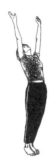

11. INHALE up to **2**. Keep your arms beside your ears so that your hands and head come up together

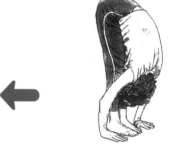

10. EXHALE the left foot forwards. Straighten the knees and bring your chest towards your thighs, coming into **Standing Forward Bend**.

Introduction

THERE ARE many different versions of the **Sun Salutations.** Most share a few similarities. The second position is upward, resembling a salutation. Most contain a **Dog**, **Cobra** or **Plank**.

It is often used at the beginning of a posture session to warm up the body and loosen the spine, with each posture counteracting the one before. The chest is alternately contracted and expanded, giving a very obvious breathing pattern.

Notes

1. In **Sun Salutations** you do not hold the postures and breathe. You make each movement with an inhalation or exhalation.
2. The hands stay in the same place between **3** and **10**.
3. Some people do not need to put the knee to the floor in **9**.

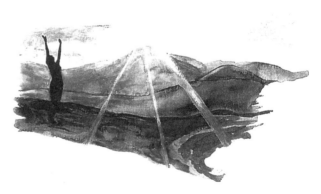

In India this sequence is traditionally practised at sunrise and sunset

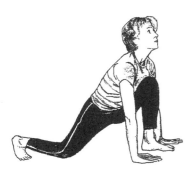
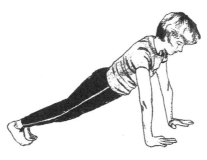
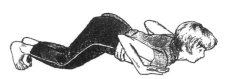

4. INHALE as you bring your right leg back and place your knee on the floor. Look up and hold your breath in preparation for **5**.

5. While retaining the breath, bring your left leg back, coming into the **Plank**. Keep your head and body in line. Look downwards.

6. EXHALE as you lower your knees, chest and chin or forehead to the floor. Your hips remain off the floor.

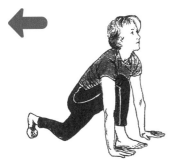
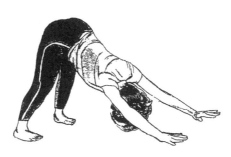
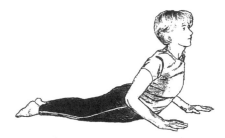

9. Lower your left knee to the floor. **INHALE** the right foot forwards so that your fingers are in line with your toes. Look up.

8. Tuck your toes under and **EXHALE** into **Downward Dog**. With straight knees, push the heels down to the floor. Move the hips backwards and sink the spine between the shoulder blades downwards. Feel the rib cage expanding.

7. INHALE as you slide forwards into **Cobra**, without moving the knees. Flatten your feet to the floor. Move the shoulders down and back and bring your elbows into your sides.

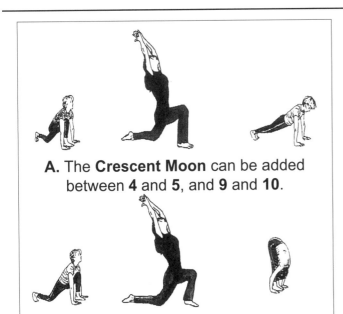

A. The **Crescent Moon** can be added between **4** and **5**, and **9** and **10**.

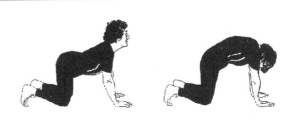

C. Pregnant women, or those with weak wrists or shoulder problems, can substitute **5**, **6** and **7**, with variations of the **Cat**, as found in the **Cat Sequence**.

Variations

Here are some variations I have come across in other yoga teachers' classes.

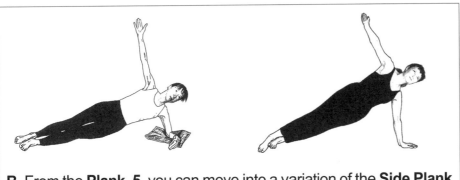

B. From the **Plank**, **5**, you can move into a variation of the **Side Plank**.

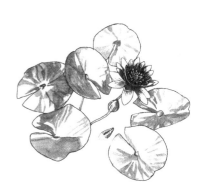

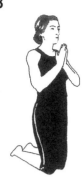

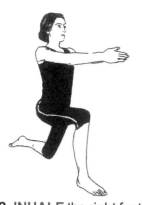

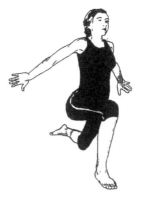

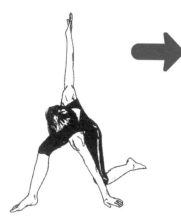

1. Kneel with the hands in **Prayer**.

2. INHALE the right foot forwards. **EXHALE** the hands forwards.

3. INHALE the hands back.

4. EXHALE the left hand to the floor. Look up at your right hand.

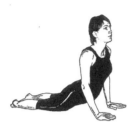

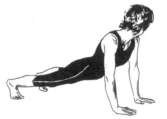

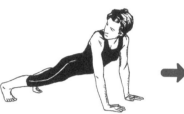

21. INHALE as you swing forwards into **Striking Cobra**. The knees do not move.

22. Go up on your toes. **EXHALE** as you twist round to the left, looking over your shoulder at the left foot.

23. INHALE the head forwards and **EXHALE** as you twist round to the right.

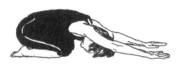

20. EXHALE the right foot down and lower the knees to the floor. **INHALE** as you lower the hips to the heels and **EXHALE** as you stretch the hands forwards, coming into **Extended Child's Pose**.

Salutations to the Moon

Introduction

FOR MOST of this sequence, similar to **Sun Salutations**, you do not hold the postures and breathe. The movement is on each inhalation and each exhalation. An exception could be made in the **Comet** posture, **12** and **14**. You could adopt a less structured breathing practice here.

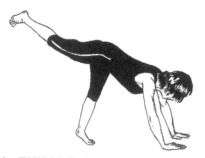

19. EXHALE the left foot down and **INHALE** the right foot up.

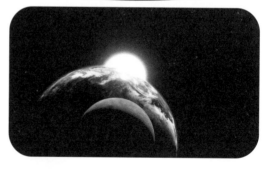

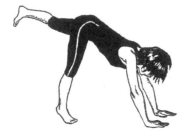

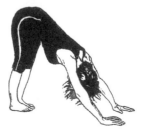

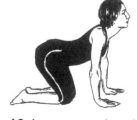

18. INHALE as you lift your left leg. The right heel can come off the floor.

17. EXHALE into **Downward Dog**.

16. Lower your hands to the floor and **INHALE** into **Upward Cat**. The spine sinks downwards. Look up.

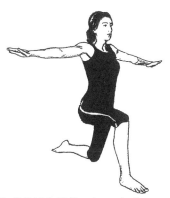

5. INHALE the hands to a central position.

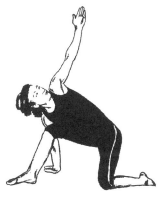

6. EXHALE the right hand to the floor. Look up at the left hand.

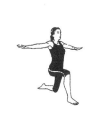

7. INHALE back to **5**.

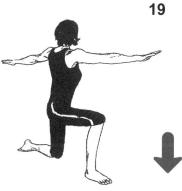

8. EXHALE as you twist round to the left.

9. INHALE back to **5**.

24. Return to **21**.

25. Return to **20**.

26. Return to **17**.

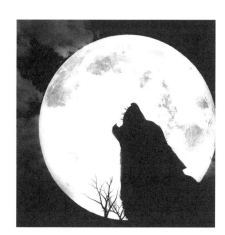

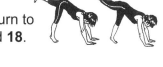

27. Return to **19** and **18**.

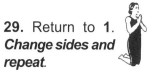

28. Return to **16**.

29. Return to **1**. *Change sides and repeat*.

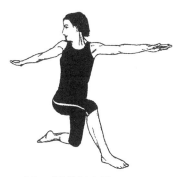

10. EXHALE as you twist round to the right.

11. INHALE back to **5**.

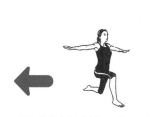

15. INHALE back to **5**.

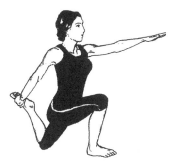

14. EXHALE your right hand to your left foot. **INHALE** your left hand forward.

13. INHALE back to **5**.

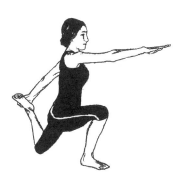

12. Lift your left foot. **EXHALE** your left hand to your right foot. **INHALE** the right hand forwards coming into the **Comet**.

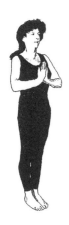 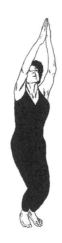 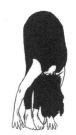

1. Stand, with the hands in **Prayer** at the **Heart Centre**. Bring your awareness to the **Heart Centre.**

2. Bend the knees. **INHALE** the hands into the **Upward Armchair.** Look at your hands and bring your awareness to the **Throat Centre.**

3. EXHALE as you lower the hands into **Standing Forward Bend**. You may keep the knees bent or straighten them. Bring your awareness to the **Solar Plexus** in the abdomen.

Varanasi Sun Salutations

Introduction

I WAS taught this powerful sequence by Sunil Kumar. I had the good fortune to study with him for one week in Varanasi in November 2004. I have inevitably added my own interpretation to it, e.g. names of postures and breathing instructions.

Attitudes and ideas about Chakras and Energy Centres vary greatly[1]. However, most people seem to find concentrating and mentally breathing into these strategic parts of the body highly beneficial.

This is a good sequence for building up **Prana** (cosmic energy) within the body. You can vary the speed you do it from very slow, holding the postures for a long time, to very fast. Sunil suggested that, after doing a few rounds, we finished up doing the whole sequence in one breath!

Sunil was exposed to yoga from a young age. His grandfather wrote a book about yoga. He called this sequence **Integrated Sun Salutations.** I have named it after Varanasi as the city and the Ganges made such a strong impression on me.

1. *I found* Energetic Anatomy *by Mark Rich very helpful. It is published by Wave of the Future, Inc. ISBN: 0-9749271-0-4*

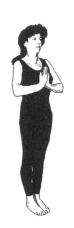 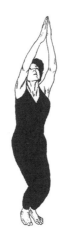 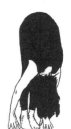

11. Return to **1**.
Repeat, changing sides on 4 and 8. This will complete one round.

10. Return to **2**.

9. Return to **3**.

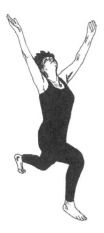

4. INHALE up. **EXHALE** as you step backwards with your left foot into **High Crescent Moon**. Both knees are bent and your back knee is off the floor. Stretch out the arms wide. Straighten the elbows and stretch to the ends of every finger. Open up the **Heart Centre** and bring your awareness to the **Third Eye** (the point between the eyebrows).

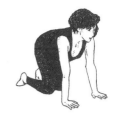
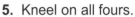

5. Kneel on all fours.

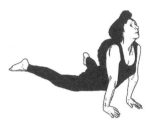

6. Widen the knees and slide the legs out to the side. Swing forwards onto the hands, coming up into a **High Cobra.** The pubic bone can just touch the floor but the abdomen is off the floor. Bring your awareness to the **Heart Centre**.

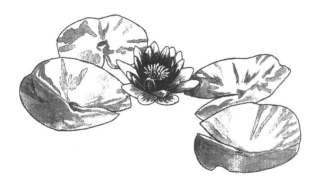

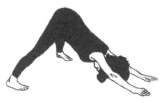

7. EXHALE as you swing back into a **Long Wide Dog**.
Sink the chest down to the floor and push the hips backwards. Bring your awareness to the **Solar Plexus** in the abdomen.

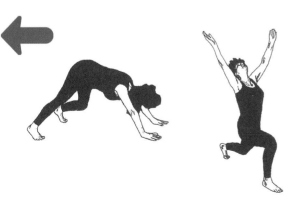

8. Move the left foot into the centre and **INHALE** as you move your right foot forwards into another **High Crescent Moon**. Bring your awareness to the **Third Eye**.

The Crescent Moon Sequence

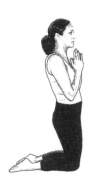

1. Kneel on the back of your mat with the hands in **Prayer**.

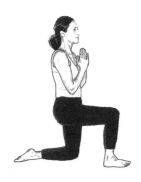

2. INHALE the right foot forwards.

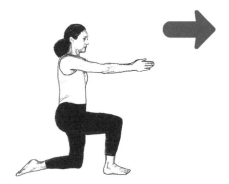

3. EXHALE the hands forwards.

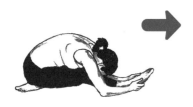

15. Sit back on your right foot, adjusting its position if necessary. **EXHALE** as you lower your head towards the straight knee. Your hands can hold your feet or ankles.

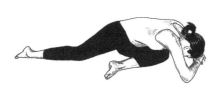

16. Bend your left knee and place it across the mat. Slide your right foot as far back as you can, straightening the leg. Lie down on top of your left leg, stretching the thigh and coming into **Sleeping Swan**. You can either rest your head on your hands or stretch your hands away in front and lower your head to the floor.

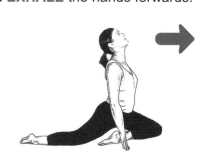

17. INHALE your head up and place your fingertips on the floor. Walk the straight arms back as far as they will go until you are leaning backwards.

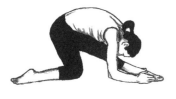

14. EXHALE your head and hands forwards. Place one hand on either side of your front leg. Move the hips backwards and straighten the leg. Bend your elbows and lower your head to your knee.

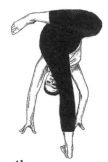

Suggestion
For a variation, when you get to **12** the second time, you can look under your left armpit at your right foot.
Change sides and repeat until 20.

Introduction

*Over the years I have expanded the basic sequence which is from **1** to **9** practised on both sides.*

*After this, I repeat the sequence adding **Dragon Wings** after the **Crescent Moon**, bending the raised leg, as in **12**, and adding **14** to **20**.*

*The complete sequence involves bending backwards into the **Crescent Moon** eight times. As your body warms up during this practice, your back will become more flexible. You will then notice that your back bends become more comfortable.*

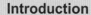

13. Swing back as before, onto your right knee and repeat **8** and **11** with the left foot forwards.

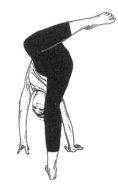

12. Swing forwards as before, into **5**. For a variation you can bend the left knee and swing the hip, leg and foot over to the right. You can push up on your left fingertips and look up under your left armpit. ***Change sides and repeat.***

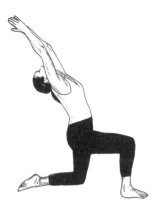

4. INHALE back into the **Crescent Moon.**

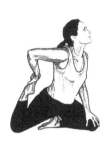

18. Bring you left heel under your left thigh. Catch hold of your right foot with your right hand and squeeze the heel towards the buttock. Place your left hand on your knee or the floor coming into the **Half Pigeon**.

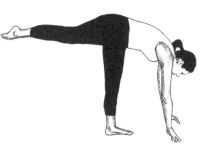

5. EXHALE as you swing forwards, placing the hands on the floor. **INHALE** as you lift your left leg.
Both knees should be straight and the balance even on both hands. You may go up on finger tips if it is more comfortable. Push your heel up towards the ceiling.

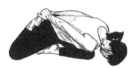

19. If you feel secure, you can place both hands on the right foot and lower your head to the floor.
Return to 9 and rest for a few breaths before changing sides and repeating from 10 onwards.

20. **Return to **9 and rest.

6. Change legs, **EXHALING** the left leg down and **INHALING** the right leg up.

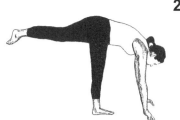

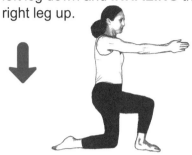

7. Lower your right knee to the floor. It needs to be as far away from the left heel as possible. Stretch your hands forwards in **Prayer**. This is the same as **3** but with the left foot forwards.

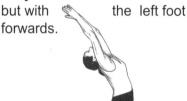

8. INHALE back into **Crescent Moon.**

9. Bring your left knee back and rest for a few breaths in **Extended Child Pose**. Your knees can be apart and the feet touching. Sink your hips down to your heels, stretching the lower spine. Let the spine between the shoulder blades relax towards the floor.
Change sides and repeat.

When you repeat **5** and **6** you can flex and point the foot a few times.

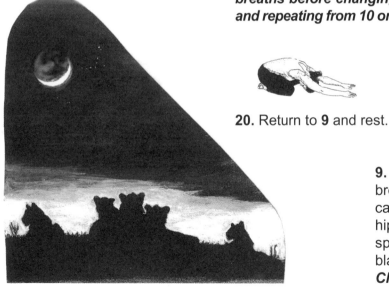

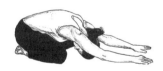

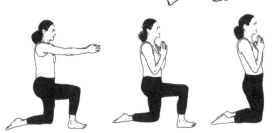

11. Separate your hands and squeeze your shoulder blades together coming into **Dragon Wings**.
Lean backwards as far as you comfortably can with the palms of your hands facing the ceiling.

10. After resting again in **Extended Child's Pose**, repeat **1, 2, 3** and **4**.

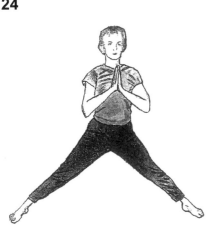

1. Stand with the legs wide and the hands in **Prayer**. Roll over onto the outsides of your feet.

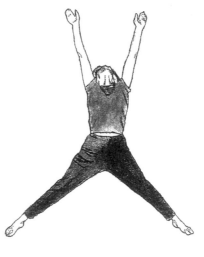

2. INHALE the hands up and back. Look up.

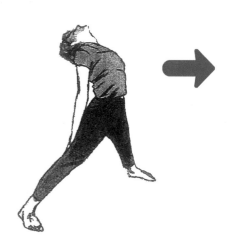

3. EXHALE your hands to the back of your thighs and lean backwards, sliding the hands down the thighs. Expand the chest forwards and squeeze the shoulder blades together.

Hero Sequence

13. Return to **1** (above).
Repeat, changing sides from 7 onwards.

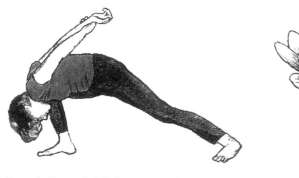

12. Bend the right knee and **EXHALE** forwards into a **Deep Lunge**. Lift the hands as high as you can and lower the head and shoulders down the inside of the right leg.

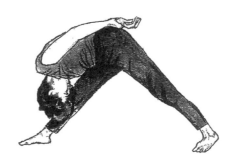

11. INHALE the head up and **EXHALE** as you lower it to the straight right knee.

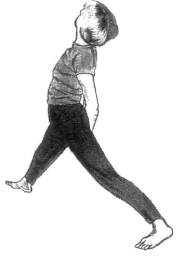

10. INHALE as you lift the head and straighten the right leg. Bring your hands behind your back and catch hold of the right wrist with the left hand. **EXHALE** as you lean backwards and slide the hands down the hips.

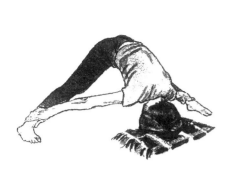

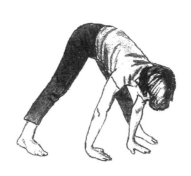

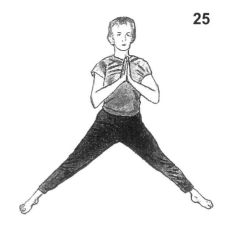

4. INHALE the head up and **EXHALE** as you slide your hands down your legs and lower the head to the floor. You will need to slide your feet further apart.

For an easier version place your hands on the floor, bend the elbows and lower the head as far as you can.

5. Place your hands on the floor and bring the feet a little closer together.

6. Soften the knees and return to **1**.

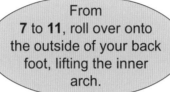

From **7** to **11**, roll over onto the outside of your back foot, lifting the inner arch.

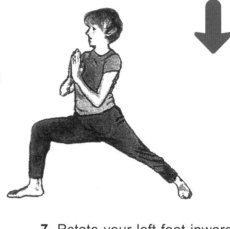

7. Rotate your left foot inwards and your right foot at a right angle. Bend your right knee. The knee should be above the ankle. Try and get the thigh parallel to the floor. Rotate over the right leg.

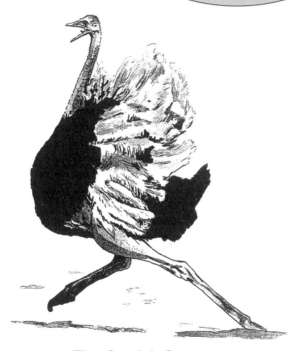

The Ostrich Strut

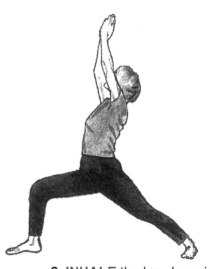

8. INHALE the hands up into the **Warrior**. Look up at your hands with the chest forwards and the arms back. Roll over onto the outside of the back foot. The hands can be together or separate.

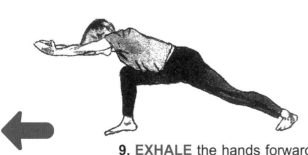

9. EXHALE the hands forwards and down. Shake the legs out at this point if you need to.

Introduction to the Figure of Eight Sequence

THIS WAS a very pleasant surprise from Bob Camp that arrived by courtesy of the British Mail.

After I had tried it out in class, one of my pupils, a teacher, said she uses **Figures of Eight** to improve the behaviour of difficult pupils. She got the idea from a pamphlet from Brain Gym she found in the staff room. I Googled 'Brain Gym, figure of eight'. Here are some quotes from their websites.

> *Rhythmic 8's energetically integrate the right and left hemispheres of the brain and will bring balance.* - Donna Eden

All other quotations are by Nancy Mramor, Ph.D.
> *... Brain Gym, a system of kinesiology developed by Paul Dennison, Ph.D., a California-based educator.*

> *Brain Gym consists of twenty-six exercises which bring attention away from the survival centres in the brain and promote better functioning.*

> *When you observe students and see them writing with their heads tipped down, one side almost to the table, they are processing information with only one hemisphere of the brain.*

> *Brain Gym uses exercises that create the conditions for:*
> *Focusing; the ability to coordinate the back and front parts of the brain.*
> *Centring; coordinating the top and bottom parts of the brain.*
> *Laterality; the ability to coordinate one side of the brain with the other.*

They say about the **Cross Crawl** exercise; *It stimulates the motor and sensory cortexes, increasing communication across the hemispheres of the brain.* Making the **Figure of Eight** has the same effect. You can practise the **Cross Crawl** sitting or standing. You can touch the opposite knee with the hand or elbow.

When I asked Malcolm Bray if he would model **Cross Crawl** for me, he said Warrior Yoga had its own variations of the same crossing movements. These can be found in the **Turtle Variations, Variation 7**.

The **Figure of Eight** has been given special significance in India and China for centuries. The Egyptians had mixed feelings about it. This is a quote from the *Encyclopaedia of Numbers* by A. E. Abbot.

> *Esotericism sees the 8 as signifying a resurrection into the higher consciousness, and represents the eternal and spiral motion of cycles. The crossing-point of the figure of 8 suggests the crossing point from earthly life to the spiritual world.*

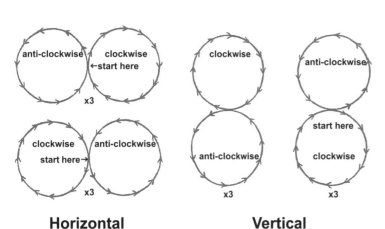

Horizontal   **Vertical**

The Eight Sequence
(Three times each way or 3+3)

Sitting: -

Eyes,
Head central, look to right, keeping the head looking to front let the eyes describe a horizontal figure 8, 3+3.
A vertical figure 8 can follow.

NECK,

Turn head to right and keeping shoulders square to the front describe a horizontal figure 8 with the chin. 3+3
Same again but with a vertical Figure 8. 3+3

SHOULDERS

Imagining a vertical egg in your shoulders describe a figure 8. 3+3. Same again but with a horizontal egg.

CAT

Lean forward and describe a figure 8 coming right back on the ankles. 3+3.

STANDING

Describe horizontal Figure 8. with hips 3+3

Hands on knees Describe a figure 8 with knees 3+3

Lift knee and describe a figure 8 with foot 3+3.
Then other foot.

I follow this with the Swimming Dragon.

Bob
October 2008

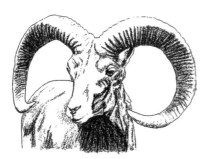

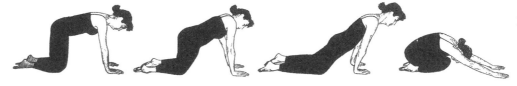

Eyes

1. Sit or stand. Look straight ahead and find a comfortable position for your chin. The head should not move.
Make an **8** with your eyes. This can be done horizontally or vertically and at least 3 times in each direction.
For clarification please refer to the diagram on the previous page.

Cat

4. Start in **Neutral Cat** with the spine flat like a table top. You can just let the spine do what it wants to do once you start moving. Following the vertical diagram, first make a clockwise circle and then continue. **Repeat three times in each direction.**
Go as far forwards and backwards as you comfortably can.

Figure of Eight Sequence

Neck

2. Sit or stand with the shoulders facing straight ahead. They should not move. Make an **8** with your chin.
Horizontal: **Repeat three times in each direction.**
Vertical: **Repeat three times in each direction.**

Symbol
8 will be used for Figure of Eight.

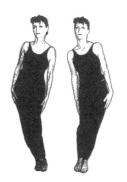

Standing
5. Hips
Make a horizontal **8** with your hips.
Repeat three times in each direction.

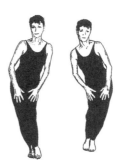

6. Knees
With your knees bent and soft, make a horizontal **8** with your knees.
Repeat three times in each direction.

Shoulders

3. You can sit or stand.
If you decide to stand, it is most enjoyable with the feet apart and the knees bent and very loose and soft.
You can make maximum use of your space and this creates a pleasant lolloping feeling.
For the horizontal version, keep the shoulders parallel to the floor.
For the vertical version, you can move parallel to the wall and go right up on your toes, then sink down as low as you can.

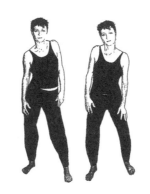
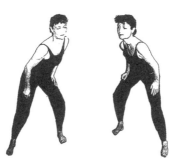
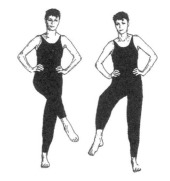

7. Feet
Lift the right knee and make an **8** with the raised foot. Do it horizontally, parallel to the floor at first. **Repeat three times in each direction.**
Change sides and repeat.
Return to right side and try it vertically, parallel to the wall. Lift the foot in front as high as you can. **Repeat three times in each direction.**
Change sides and repeat.

The Five Tibetan Rites

I CAN'T do justice to this dynamic sequence in two pages. I read about them in a little booklet called *The Eye of Revelation*[1] by Peter Kelder. It is no longer available from bookshops. In addition to practising the Five Rites every day, they chewed their food until it was liquid, ate one raw egg yolk a day and did not mix their food types. *The Ancient Secrets of the Fountain of Youth*[2] contains the necessary background information. It is also available on the Internet.

The more recent publications use the yogic chakra system to position the vortexes. Their interpretation of the original drawings of the postures differ slightly from mine.

Peter Kelder met Colonel Bradford (a pseudonym) before he went back to India to trace a particular Tibetan monastery and to discover the Fountain of Youth. The Colonel was in his late 60s, was thin and stooped and walked with a cane. When he returned a few years later however, Peter Kelder thought the man he saw approaching must be the Colonel's son because he looked so much younger and was walking without a stick. Peter Kelder is the only source of information about the Five Rites.

The position of the seven vortexes (electro-magnetic energy centres).
A. In the forehead; B. The back of the head; C. The throat; D. Above the waist on the right side of the body; E. The reproductive organs; F. & G. One in each knee.

In a healthy person, the vortexes extend outside the body and all spin at the same speed. As they diminish and spin at different speeds, we become old. To stay young we need to keep them spinning. This is the function of the Five Rites.

The Buddhist Lamas advised that Rites 2-5 should each be practised 21 times a day. You pace this according to your level of fitness. You could start with seven times for a few days and then try 11 times and slowly build up until you can manage 21 times. You would start each practice with Rite Number 1 and the Lamas advised that you only rotate 12 times ... until you feel comfortable and familiar with the practice.

When you practise the Five Rites you will feel the benefits quickly. The action of the chin and neck in Rites 2-5 is a particular feature of this sequence. It is similar to Jalandhara Bandha[3]. It cannot fail to affect the thyroid gland and release tension in that area. Those with speech problems, public speakers and singers in particular could expect to benefit from this practice.

There is a sixth rite, but it is for committed celibates only. It involves directing sexual energy up the spine. It is not usually included in yoga classes.

1. *© 1939 by Peter Kelder & 1975 by Borderlands Sciences Research Foundation.*
2. *© 1985 Published by Doubleday.*
3. *This is described at the beginning of* The Four Directions.

Rite Number One

This is the Swirling Dervish, as practised by many different sects, including Christian and mystic Muslim, throughout the world.
Stand with the arms out to the sides, parallel to the floor. Spin around clockwise, from left to right.
Whereas some sects would spin for hours, the Lamas advised only about 12 rounds at first. Too many spins at first has a counterproductive effect on the vortexes.

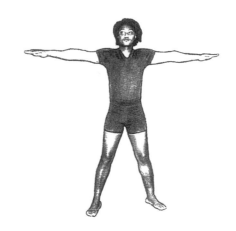

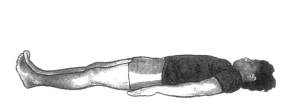
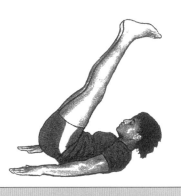

Rite Number Two - Make sure the spine is well cushioned with a thick mat. Lie on your back with the arms by your sides. Move the hands a little under your hips. Turn the fingers slightly inwards. Press down with the palms and lift the legs up, keeping the knees straight. At the same time lift the head and shoulders up and tuck in the chin. Bring the legs over your head and, if you can, lift the hips off the floor.

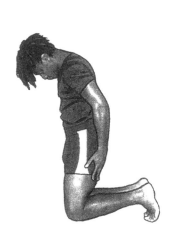
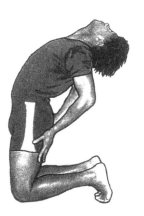
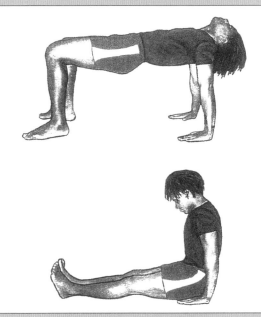

Rite Number Three

Proceed immediately after practising Rite Number Two. Kneel on your mat, knees together and hands on the back of the thighs. Go up on your toes.

Lean forwards as much as you can, without moving the hips backwards. Tuck in the chin.

Now lean backwards and let your head fall backwards if it is comfortable. This Rite speeds up vortexes C, D and E in particular.

Rite Number Four - If you find this Rite difficult, persevere unless there is a physical problem, and slowly build up the practice. Sit on your mat with the feet stretched out in front, toes pointing forwards and your hands beside your hips. Tuck your chin in to your chest. Now raise your body, bending the knees and pushing up on the hands.

The arms and lower legs should be at right angles to the floor. The rest of the body should be parallel to the floor, like a table top. The head can fall gently backwards, stretching the neck and throat. When you have established the position, tense all the muscles of the body, including the pelvic floor.

This Rite speeds up vortexes C, E, F and G in particular.

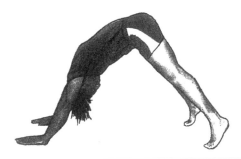
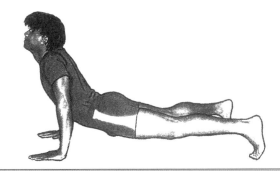

Rite Number Five - Position yourself face downwards with the hands and feet at least a shoulder-width apart, (the book says two feet apart). Tuck the toes under. Push up on your toes and hands and lift the hips as high as possible. Tuck the chin into the chest. After establishing the posture, tense all your muscles and then lower the body down to a 'sagging position'. You will need to experiment with the placing of your hands and feet so that you can move up and down without moving them. The knees should be low but not touching the floor. Look up and stretch the front of your neck. At your lowest point, tense all your muscles.

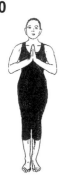
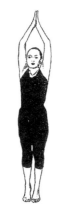
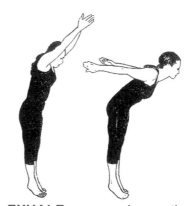
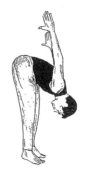

1. Stand with the feet together and the hands in **Prayer.**

2. INHALE up onto tiptoes and lift the hands above your head.

3. EXHALE as you lower the head with the chin forwards. Swing the hands back in **Flying Bird**. Balance for a few breaths in the **Divers Posture**.

4. If you feel confident, look at your knees. Lower the chin and stretch the back of your neck.

Diver's Posture Sequence

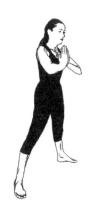

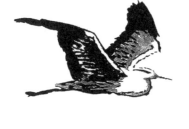

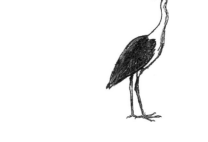

21. INHALE as you stand upright. **EXHALE** the hands into **Prayer**.

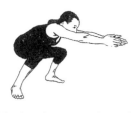

20. Look up and push away with your hands.

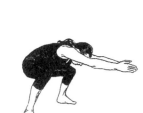

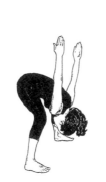

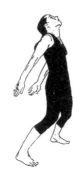

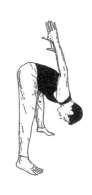

19. Lower the arms. Look down and sink into a deeper squat.

18. When you are ready, sink down into a deep squat and swing the hands up high.

17. Lower the heels to the floor, bend the knees and lean backwards. Close your eyes and hold as in **6**.

16. Lower the head as far as you can and, if you feel confident, look behind you.

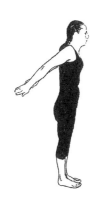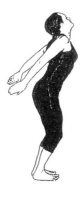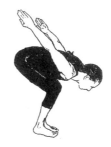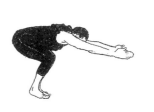

5. **EXHALE** the heels to the floor.

6. Bend the knees and lean backwards, with the chin lifted if it is comfortable. Squeeze the shoulder blades together and expand the chest forwards. Close your eyes and hold for a few breaths.

7. Deepen the squat and lower the head. Look down and lift the hands as high as you can.

8. **INHALE** as you stretch the hands out in front. Separate the palms and sink into a deeper squat.

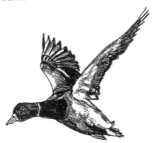

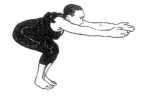

9. Look up and push away with the hands.

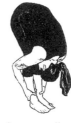

10. When you are ready, **EXHALE** as you straighten the knees and catch hold of your ankles.

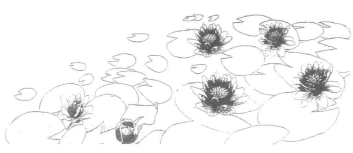

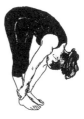

11. Bend your elbows and bring the head towards the knees. Hold and breathe in the **Standing Forward Bend.**

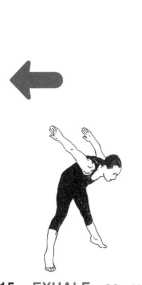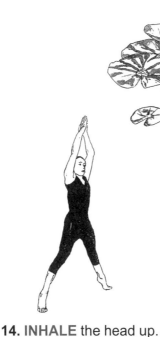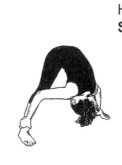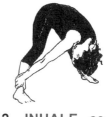

15. **EXHALE** as you lower the head, with the chin forwards, and swing your hands back in **Flying Bird**. This is the **Wide Diver's Posture**.

14. **INHALE** the head up. Go up on tiptoes again and lift the hands above your head in **Prayer**. We now repeat from **1** to **12** with the feet wide apart.

13. **EXHALE** as you bend the elbows and pull your head through the knees.

12. **INHALE** as you widen your stance and look behind you.

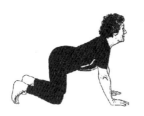

1. Kneel on all fours with the hands under the shoulders. The feet can be flat or raised on the toes.
INHALE as you curve the lower spine downwards and look up. Stretch the front of the neck and lift the chin.
This curvature of the spine is called the **Dog Tilt**.

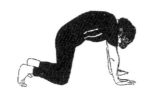

2. EXHALE as you lower the head and arch the spine upwards. Push up on your hands.
Tuck the tail bone in and tighten the abdomen. This curvature is called the **Cat Tilt**.
Do this three times.

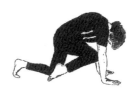

3. INHALE and then **EXHALE** as you swing the right knee forwards. Try and get your forehead to your knee.

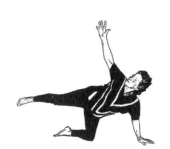

7. Turn your fingers forwards again. Lift your right leg and hand, and look up, coming into **Balancing Cat**.
Hold for a few breaths.

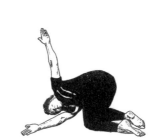

8. Go straight into the **Cat's Paw Stretch**.*
Lower your right leg and place the back of your right hand on the floor. Slide it to the left and lower your right shoulder and head to the floor. Lift your left hand up and bring your left shoulder back.

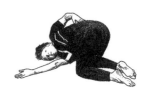

9. Lower your left hand to your hip and twist around more.
Please note: Some people will feel quite comfortable with their shoulder on the floor and the head tilted sideways.
Others will not get their shoulder to the floor and may prefer to rest nearer the top of the head. Some experimentation may be necessary.
Change sides and repeat 7, 8 and 9.

The Cat Sequence

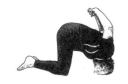

13. Roll over onto the back of your head coming into the **Cat Neck Stretch**.*
This stretches the back of your neck and tucks in your chin. Hold for a few breaths.
Caution: Avoid this posture if you have neck problems.

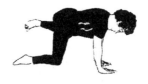

14. Return to **Neutral Cat**.
INHALE as you lift the right knee coming into **Rovers Revenge**. Keep the knee tightly bent and the balance even on both hands. Lift the knee as high as you can. **EXHALE** the knee down.
Do this three times.

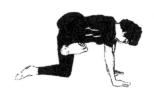

15. After you have lifted the knee for the third time, straighten out the leg to the side.
Push the sole of the foot away and lift the leg as high as you can. Hold for a few breaths.

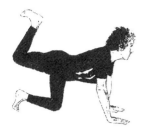 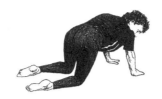 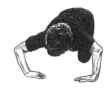

4. INHALE as you swing the leg back. Keep it bent and push the sole of your foot towards the ceiling.
Do this three times.

5. Come into a **Neutral Cat**, with a *table top* back. **INHALE.** As you **EXHALE**, swing your hips to the right and look over your right shoulder into **Cat looks at its Tail.** The spine is in a **C** shape and the left side of your neck is stretched.
Do this three times, then change sides and repeat.

6. Turn your fingers to face each other and soften the elbows. Bend your right elbow and swing your hips to the left coming into **Sideways Cat.**
Hold for a few breaths pushing your right elbow away from the left hip.
Change sides and repeat.

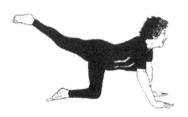 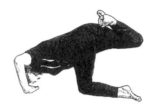 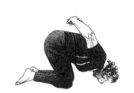

10. Return to **3**. And then straighten your leg as you swing it back and point your toes.
Hold for a few breaths, looking up and lifting the leg up high.

11. Turn your fingers towards each other and lower the head to the floor.
Lift your leg as high as you can. Bend your right leg and swing it over to the left. Look up under your left armpit at your right foot. Hold for a few breaths.

12. Lower your leg and find a comfortable position for your head on the floor. Interlock the fingers behind your head and push away with your palms.

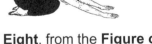

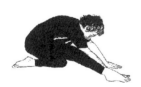

16. Swing the leg round to the outside of your right arm. Straighten the leg and place the toes on the floor. Slowly lower the hips back and down coming into the **Backward Cat**. Feel the stretch on the back of the right leg. Hold for a few breaths.

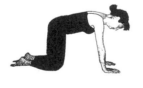 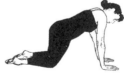 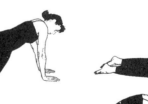

17. To conclude, you can do **Cat in Figure of Eight**, from the **Figure of Eight Sequence**.
Make a clockwise circle, going as far forwards as you comfortably can, and then an anti-clockwise circle backwards, going as far back as you can.
Do this three times, then change sides and repeat.

18. Rest in **Extended Child's Pose.**

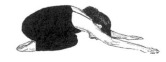

＊ *The Cat's Paw Stretch is sometimes called Threading the Needle and the Cat Neck Stretch, the Hare. I have changed their names to avoid confusion.*

The Cat Sequence (continued)

With some modification you can do this sequence holding on to the seat of a chair, or to a secure support about the same height as the back of a chair. This makes an interesting sequence in its own right and is also helpful for somebody with bad knees. Here are some examples:

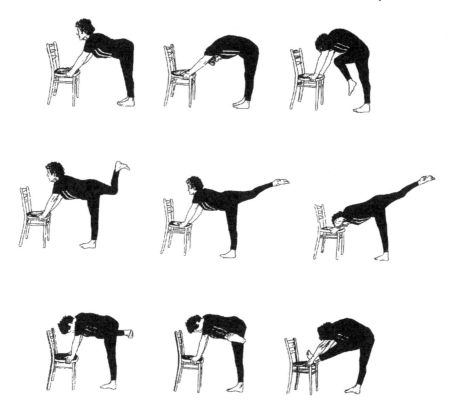

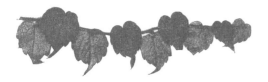

Taoist Meditation

Close your eyes and you will see clearly

Cease to listen and you will hear the truth

Be silent and your heart will sing

Seek no contacts and you will find union

Be still and you will move forward

on the tide of the spirit

You are all little flowers
Swami Sivananda

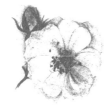

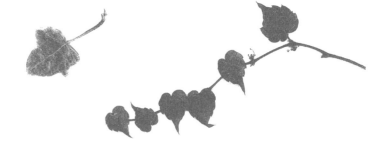

Quotations from Albert Einstein

Reality is merely an illusion,
albeit a very persistent one.

The only valuable thing is intuition.

All religions, arts and sciences
are branches of the same tree.

Science without religion is lame.
Religion without science is blind.

The only thing that interferes with my learning
is my education.

Few are those who see with their eyes
and feel with their hearts.

Imagination is more important than knowledge.

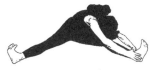

IF YOU suffer from sciatic pain due to a trapped nerve, you may be lucky and un-trap it with these stretches. Two of my pupils found immediate pain relief when they did **5** for the first time.

1. Sit with the legs wide apart. Bring the toes back towards the head. Rotate over the left leg. **INHALE** the hands up. **EXHALE** as you slide the hands along the leg as far as you can.

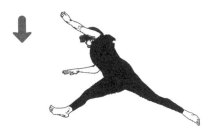

2. INHALE as you swing over onto your right elbow and stretch your left hand over your head. First push away with your left heel for a few breaths and then point your toes to increase the stretch. Push away on the exhalations.
Change sides and repeat.

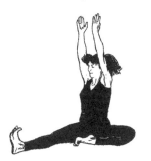

3. Place your left foot along your right thigh. Rotate over your right leg. **INHALE** the hands up.

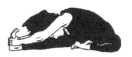

4. EXHALE the hands down to the foot or the lower leg. Bend your elbows and bring your head forwards and down.

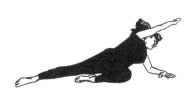

5. INHALE as you swing over onto your left elbow and stretch your right hand over your head. Look down at the floor. Bring your right foot back a little, point your toes and stretch along your right side in the **Sciatic Stretch**.

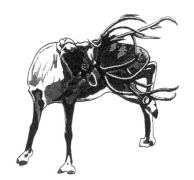

Reindeer Itch
A reindeer uses its antlers
to scratch a back leg.

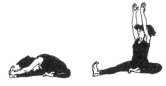

6. Return to **3** and **4**.

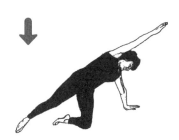

7. INHALE as you swing over to the left as in **5**, but this time onto your left hand instead of the elbow. Continue as in **5**.

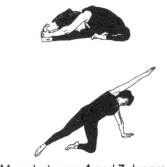

8. Move between **4** and **7** dynamically. **INHALE** into **7** and **EXHALE** into **4**. Repeat about six times.
Change sides and repeat.

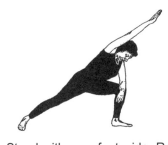

9. Stand with your feet wide. Rotate your left foot at a right angle and turn your right foot in a little. **INHALE** as you bend the left knee and place the left elbow on the knee. **EXHALE** your right hand over your head. Roll over onto the outside of your back foot. Hold and breathe, pushing away on the exhalations.
Change sides and repeat.

36

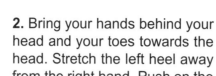
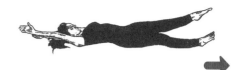

1. Lie on your back with your hands by your sides, palms facing upwards.

2. Bring your hands behind your head and your toes towards the head. Stretch the left heel away from the right hand. Push on the exhalations as described below.

3. INHALE as you lift your left foot and your right hand. Point the toes. Hold and stretch. *Change sides and repeat.*

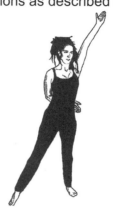
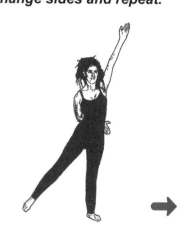

17. INHALE as you stretch the right palm upwards and the left palm downwards. This is **Heaven and Earth Stretch**. Close your eyes and hold it for as long as you want to. Keep pushing away with the palms of your hands. *Change sides and repeat from 14 to 17.*

18. Stand with the feet together. Move the right foot out to the side and point your toes. Bring your right hand behind your back. Stretch your left hand out to the side with the palm facing forwards. Push the fingers away from the toes.

19. INHALE as you lift the right foot about six inches (15 cm). Continue to stretch away.

Diagonal Stretch Sequence

A COLLEAGUE, who also teaches yoga in the field of mental health, said she had observed that her pupils find diagonal stretches very calming. She demonstrated **3**, and this led to the gradual unfolding of this sequence.

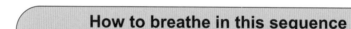

How to breathe in this sequence
All the stretches in this sequence extend on the exhalations. Get into a posture, breathe slowly, and then push across your diagonal stretch on the exhalations. Hold the posture until you feel the benefits and then release the stretch on the exhalation.

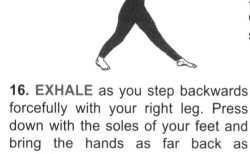

16. EXHALE as you step backwards forcefully with your right leg. Press down with the soles of your feet and bring the hands as far back as possible.

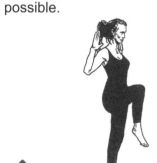
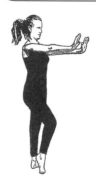
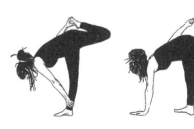

15. INHALE as you lift the right knee as high as possible and bring the hands back. Drop the shoulders and squeeze the shoulder blades together.

14. Stand with the feet together and then lift the right heel and press up on the toes. Extend the hands in front with the fingers pointing upwards. Push away with the palms of your hands.

13. When you feel ready, catch hold of the left foot with the right hand. You can either keep your left hand on the hip, lower it to the floor or catch hold of your right leg. *Change sides and repeat 12 and 13.*

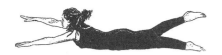

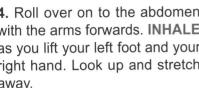

4. Roll over on to the abdomen with the arms forwards. **INHALE** as you lift your left foot and your right hand. Look up and stretch away.
Change sides and repeat.

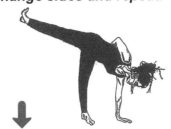

5. The Extended Bow. Catch hold of your left foot with your left hand. Stretch out your right hand. **INHALE** as you lift the left knee and the right hand. Look up and stretch away.
Change sides and repeat.

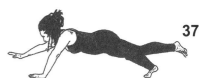

6. The Diagonal Plank. Come into the **Plank** (as described in **Salutations to the Sun** page 16). Place the hands a little closer than usual. **INHALE** as you lift your left leg and your right hand.
Change sides and repeat.

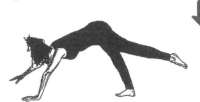

7. The Diagonal Dog. Kneel on all fours to get the right positioning of the hands and feet and then come up into the **Dog** (*see Dog Sequence page 120*). **INHALE** as you lift your left foot and right hand. You need not lift them very high. Press down with the right heel.
Change sides and repeat.

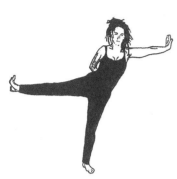

20. Turn the left palm to the left and point the toes of the right foot up to the ceiling. **INHALE** as you lift your right leg and lower the left hand.

21. Lower the hand to the floor or catch hold of the left leg. Lift the leg as high as you can.
Change sides and repeat from 18 to 21.

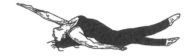

Caution: If you have a neck problem, you may choose to miss out this posture.

22. Lie on your back with your feet together and hands close by your sides. **INHALE** as you come up into the **Fish** (*see the Shoulder Stand Sequence page 68*). Lift your right leg and point your toes. Bring your left arm up and back. Hold and stretch the fingers away from the toes.
Change sides and repeat.

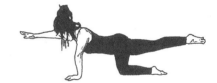

8. The Tiger Stretch. Come onto all fours again. **INHALE** as you lift your left leg and your right hand. Look down at the floor. Point your toes and stretch away with the fingers.

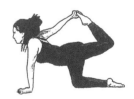

9. The Tiger Bow. Catch hold of your left foot with your right hand. Look up and lift the foot as high as possible.
Change sides and repeat 8 and 9.

> Stretches feel a little different every time you do them. They lengthen and develop with repetition and become interesting.

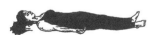

23. Return to **1**.

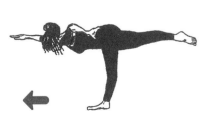

12. Come away from your support. Put your left hand on your hip. Lift your left leg and stretch away with your right hand.

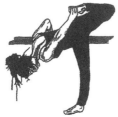

11. Catch hold of your right foot with your left hand. Lower the head and lift the knee as high as possible.
Change sides and repeat 10 and 11.

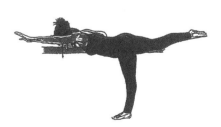

10. Stand up. Catch hold of a firm support with the right hand and stand facing sideways. **INHALE** as you lift your right leg and your left hand. Look down and push the toes away from the fingers.

Abdominal Section

Leg Raises

The Jack Knife

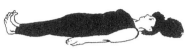

1. Lie on your back with your hands close to your sides and palms facing downwards. Push the shoulders down towards your feet.

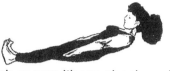

2. Push away with your heels and bring your toes towards your head.
Without lifting your feet, **INHALE** your shoulders, arms and upper body off the floor. Hold and breathe.

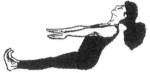

3. INHALE up into the **Jack Knife**. Lean backwards and push the hands forward. The head can fall back if it is comfortable.

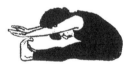

4. EXHALE the hands over the feet. See how far forwards your hands will go without touching the feet.

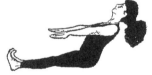

5. INHALE back into the **Jack Knife**.

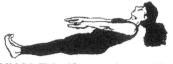

6. EXHALE half way down. Hold and breathe for as long as you comfortably can.

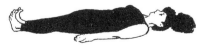

7. When you are ready, **EXHALE** back to **1**.
Repeat three times.

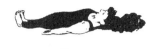

1. Lie on your back with your hands a little way from your sides and the palms facing downwards.

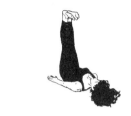

2. Press down with your palms. **INHALE** as you lift the feet up towards the ceiling.

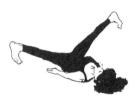

3. EXHALE the feet down to the sides.

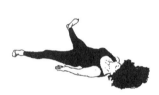

4. Swing them forwards without touching the floor.

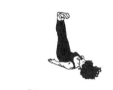

5. INHALE the legs up, returning to **2**.
Repeat three times.

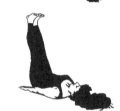

6. Sink the hollow of your back into the floor. **EXHALE** as you lower your feet about nine inches (23cm).

7. INHALE back to **2**.

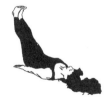

8. EXHALE the feet half way down. Hold and breathe.

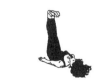

9. INHALE back to **2**.

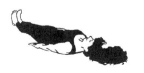

10. EXHALE your feet about three inches (8cm) off the floor. Hold and breathe.

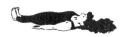

11. Lower the feet, returning to **1**.

The U Shape

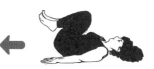

1. Lie on your back with your hands by your sides and the palms facing downwards. **INHALE** the knees up.

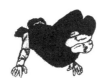

2. EXHALE the knees half way down to the left.

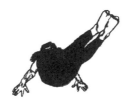

3. INHALE as you straighten the legs. Press down with the palms of your hands.

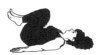

4. Return to **1**.

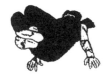

5. EXHALE the knees half way down to the right.

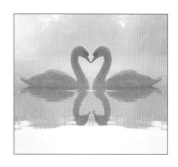

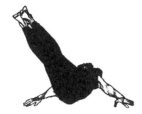

6. INHALE as you straighten the legs.

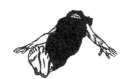

7. Make a **U** shape with your feet. **EXHALE** the feet down to the centre, keeping the knees straight and the feet off the floor.

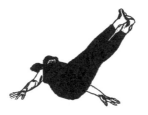

8. INHALE the feet up to the right.
*Make the **U** shape at least three times.*

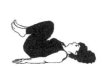

9. Return to **1**.

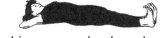

1. Lie on your back and interlock the fingers behind your head.

Cycling

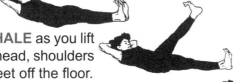

2. INHALE as you lift your head, shoulders and feet off the floor.

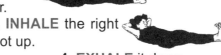

3. INHALE the right foot up.

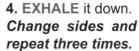

4. EXHALE it down.
Change sides and repeat three times.

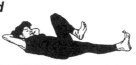

5. INHALE your right knee back.

6. EXHALE it forwards.
Change sides and repeat three times.

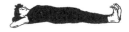

7. Return to **1**.

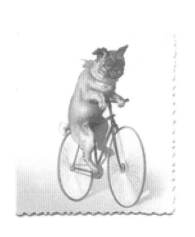

Abdominal Workout

THESE ABDOMINAL exercises come from a workshop by Zoe Knott entitled *Strength in Asana.*

1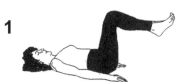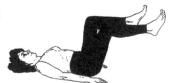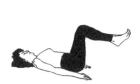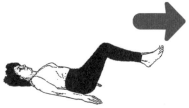

1. Lie on your back with your hands by your sides. Bend your knees with the thighs at a right angle to the floor and the lower legs parallel to the floor. Press the waist and lower back down into the floor.

2. Keep the left knee still. For the next three breaths move your right knee forward about two inches, each time you **EXHALE**. Keep the knee still when you **INHALE**. With the lower back pushed into the floor and the abdominal muscles engaged, hold the posture for about five breaths.

3. Return to **1** using the same method, moving each time you **EXHALE** until the knees are together. ***Change sides and repeat.***

4. Repeat **1** to **3** moving both knees at the same time.

2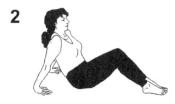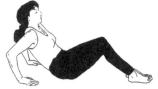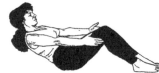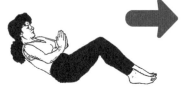

1. Sit with the legs bent in front and the arms behind, fingers pointing forward. Drop the shoulders down and back.

2. Bend the elbows and lean backwards, tucking the hips under and rounding the spine.

3. **INHALE** the arms forward. Keep the back of the neck long.

4. **EXHALE** the hands together in **Prayer**.

3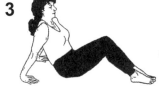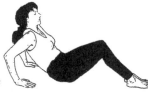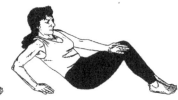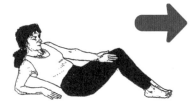

1. Sit with the legs bent in front and the arms behind, fingers pointing forward. Drop the shoulders down and back.

2. Bend the elbows and lean backwards, tucking the hips under and rounding the spine.

3. Place the back of your left hand on the outside of your right knee and twist round to the right.

4. Holding the twist, lower your right elbow down to the floor.

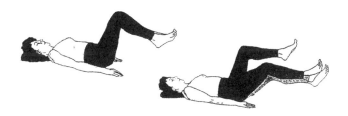 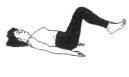 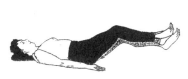

5. Return to **1**, but start with the knees a little further forward.

6. Proceed as in **2**, moving the right foot forward as you **EXHALE**. This time the foot moves further away and down until it is hovering above the floor. Hold as before.

7. Return to **5** moving on the exhalations. *Change sides and repeat.*

8. Repeat with both legs moving forward at the same time.

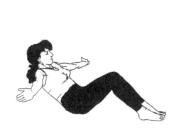 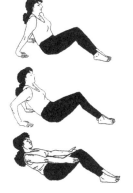 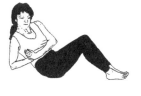 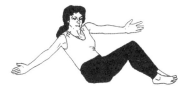

5. INHALE the hands wide apart.
Repeat 4 and 5 about five times.

6. Repeat **1**, **2** and **3**.

7. EXHALE as you twist round to the right and bring your hands into **Prayer**.

8. Hold the twist and **INHALE** the hands wide apart. Continue to hold the twist while repeating the arm movements about five times.
Change sides and repeat 7 and 8.

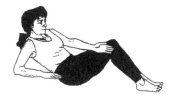 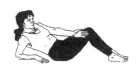 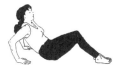 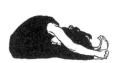

5. INHALE as you lift the elbow and hand a few inches off the floor. Let them hover there for about five breaths.

6. Return to **4**.

7. Untwist and return to **2**.

8. Release into any version of the **Sitting Forward Bend**.
Change sides and repeat.

Rock and Groove

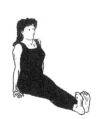

1

The Abdominal Rock.
Cross your feet over and interlock your hands behind your head. Lift your head and shoulders and bring the knees towards your head. Rock backwards and forwards.

Introduction

HERE ARE some other abdominal exercises that my pupils find beneficial.

I have arranged them in this order to form a sequence but, if you are unfit, you will need to practise two or three at a time at first. Slowly build up to include more.

Placing a blanket on top of your mat is advisable.

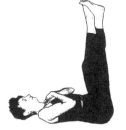

3

A. Cross the hands over on the chest and cross the feet over. Lift the legs.

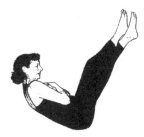

B. INHALE the head and shoulders up and rock backwards and forwards. When you are ready, return to **A**.
Place the bottom hand on top, change the feet over and repeat.

2

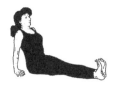

A. Sit with the legs forward, the hands by your sides and the toes towards your head. Move the shoulders down and back, slightly tuck in your chin and stretch the top of your head towards the ceiling. Observe your breathing.

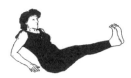

B. Move the hands further back.

C. Bend the elbows. Lean backwards and INHALE the legs up.

Sitting Balance

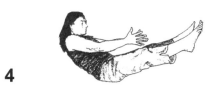

4

Start either on your back or in the **Sitting Balance**.
A. INHALE into the **Boat**.

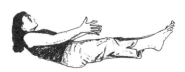

B. EXHALE half way down or into the **Sitting Balance**.
Repeat a few times.

D. EXHALE back to **B**.
Repeat three times.
The third time, hold **C** for as long as you comfortably can.

Here are some variations.

The legs and arms can be together or wide apart.
The hands can be in **Prayer** or in **Venus Lock** with the palms facing forwards.
The fists can be clenched and the hands can be in the middle or on the outsides of the legs.

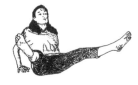

E. Proceed as above but with the hands and feet further apart. Also, when you EXHALE back, the feet can touch in the middle with the knees bent.

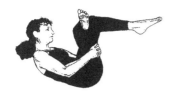

5

A. Bend your right knee and place your left foot over the right knee.
Lift the right foot. With the left hand passing through the middle, between the thighs, interlock your hands around the right thigh.
Rock backwards and forwards.

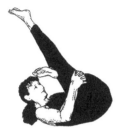

B. Straighten the right leg and point your toes. Pull the leg towards your head with your hands but push the leg in the opposite direction. This causes **dynamic tension**. Continue to rock backwards and forwards.
Change sides and repeat.

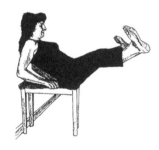

6

Find a chair or a stool with a fairly long seat. Push it against a wall. If you are tall you will need more length. Hold on to a comfortable place and lean back, resting on the wall or back of the chair.
A. INHALE the legs out to the sides and EXHALE them back a few times.

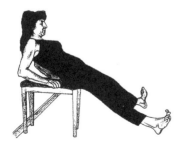

B. Make a figure of eight with your legs, moving them in opposite directions.
Swing both legs down together and then out to the sides and up.
Repeat a few times and then change direction.

7

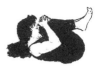

A. Hug your knees to you. Interlock the fingers on top of the knees. Bring your head towards your knees and feel the stretch on the back of your neck.
Rock backwards and forwards.

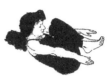

B. Remove your hands. Let them hover at your sides with the palms facing downwards. Continue rocking.

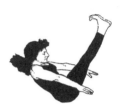

C. INHALE the legs up with the toes towards your head. Rock as vigorously as you can.
When you are ready, rest in a comfortable position.

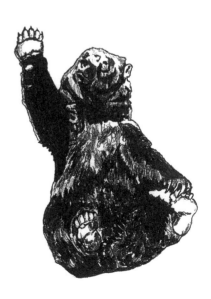

A grizzly bear having fun.

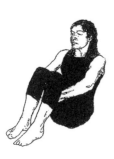

1. Clasp the fingers together, as illustrated, under the knees with the feet off the floor.

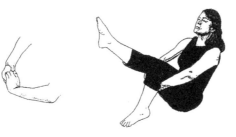

2. INHALE as you straighten the right leg.
Change sides and repeat.

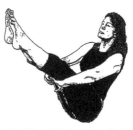

3. Straighten both legs.

Boat Balancing 1

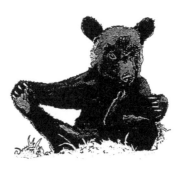

**A baby black bear experiments
with a sitting balance**

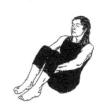

4. Return to **1.**

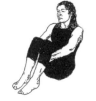

9. Return to **1.**

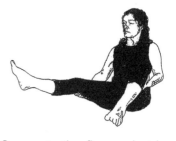

5. Separate the fingers but keep the hands under the knees. INHALE as you straighten the right leg out to the side.
Change sides and repeat.

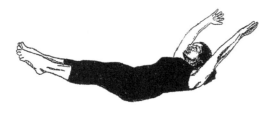

8. EXHALE as you lower the feet a little and take the arms backwards over the head. The shoulders should not touch the floor.
Repeat 7 and 8 a few times.

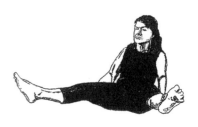

6. INHALE as you widen both legs.

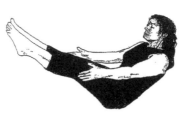

7. EXHALE the feet together. INHALE as you lift the hands and come into the **Boat**.

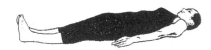

1. Lie on your back with your hands by your sides and the palms facing downwards.

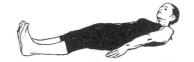

2. Push your heels away. Slide the fingers forward and **INHALE** shoulders off the floor. Keep your feet on the floor.

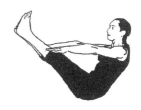

3. INHALE up into the **Boat**.

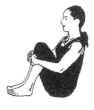

4. EXHALE into **Sitting Balance**. Keeping your feet off the floor, bend your knees and hug them tightly to you, interlocking the fingers.

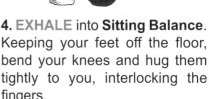

5. INHALE as you lift your legs. They should be parallel to the floor. Hold under your knees.

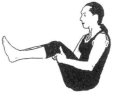

6. INHALE as you straighten the legs and arms.

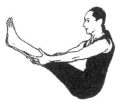

7. EXHALE into **Open Sitting Balance**. Hold onto your feet and pull them in and up, moving the knees outwards.

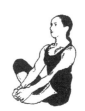

8. INHALE as you straighten the legs and arms.

16. Return to **1**.

15. Return to **3**.

14. Return to **4**.

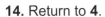
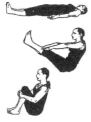

Boat Balancing 2

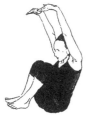

13. EXHALE the knees together into **Baby Swan**.

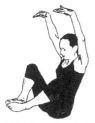

12. EXHALE the feet together, bending the knees outwards. **INHALE** the hands over the head, curving the hands forwards into **Wide Baby Swan**.

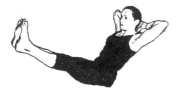

11. EXHALE the feet together, and **INHALE** the hands behind your head. Interlock the fingers and hold in the **Angular Position.**

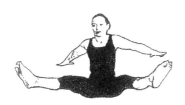

10. INHALE the hands backwards. Lower the legs and lean slightly backwards ... keeping the feet off the floor.

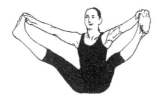

9. INHALE the legs out to the sides. Straighten the knees in the **Wide Sitting Balance**.

The Turtle Variations

THIS IS the basic Kura-Kura **Turtle** posture. From a sitting position, lift the legs and bring the heels together. The feet turn outwards and the knees widen.

The thumbs form an **L-shape** with the rest of the hands and the fingers are kept together. Cross the forearms over. This is called **Male and Female Hands**. Malcolm Bray says it doesn't matter which hand is in front. The elbows touch the knees or as high up the thigh as possible. Try to return the elbows to the knees when you move back to the posture.

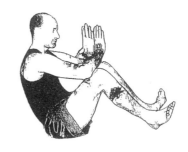
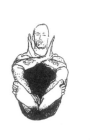

Variation 1

1. Establish the basic **Turtle** posture, as described above.

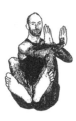

2. After a few breaths, twist the shoulders and arms round to the left. The head does not turn but continues to look straight ahead.

3. EXHALE back to **1**.

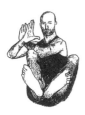

4. Repeat, twisting to the right.

5. Return to **1**.
Repeat as many times as you comfortably can.

Variation 2

1. Establish the basic **Turtle** posture.

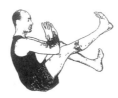

2. Make a circle with your right leg.

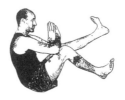

3. Make a circle with your left leg, forming a figure of eight.
Continue for as long as you comfortably can.

Variation 3

1. Establish the basic **Turtle** posture.

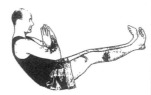

2. INHALE as you extend both legs forwards.

3. EXHALE back to **1**.
Repeat, keeping within your comfort zone.

Variation 4

This is the same as **Variation 3** except that the legs are higher.

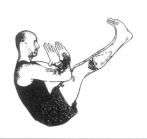

Variation 5

1. Establish the basic **Turtle** posture.

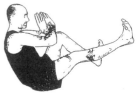

2. With the left leg bent, INHALE and extend the right leg forwards.

3. EXHALE back to **1**.

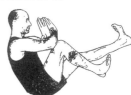

4. Change sides.
Keep the right leg bent and INHALE the left foot forwards.

5. EXHALE back to **1**.
Repeat, keeping within your comfort zone.

Variation 6

1. Establish the basic **Turtle** posture.

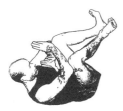

2. Rock backwards onto the right shoulder.

3. Rock back to **1**. Always bring the elbows back to the knees.

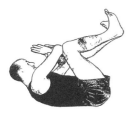

4. Rock backwards onto the left shoulder.

5. Rock back to **1**.
Repeat as before.

Variation 7

This is the Warrior Yoga equivalent of the **Cross Crawl** as taught by Brain Gym.

1. Establish the basic **Turtle** posture.

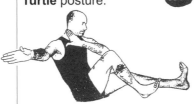

2. Bring the left elbow to the right knee. Stretch the right hand out to the side.

3. Return to **1**.

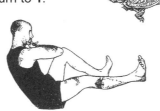

4. Bring your right elbow to your left knee and stretch your left hand out to the side.

5. Return to **1**.
Repeat as before.

Variations

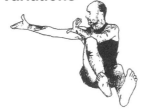

You can just keep changing from side to side, without returning to **Male and Female Hands**.
You can look forwards or look at the hand that is stretched out to the side.

Standing Cross Crawl

This is a standing Warrior Yoga version of **Cross Crawl**.

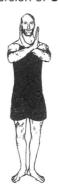

1. Stand with the heels together and the toes turned outwards. Bend your knees. Place the hands in **Male and Female** position. Remember to keep the fingers together and the thumbs in an **L-shape**.

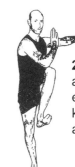

2. Lift the left knee and bring your right elbow to your left knee. Stretch the left arm out to the side.

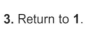

3. Return to **1**.

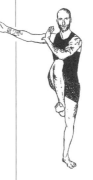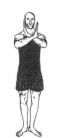

4. Change sides and repeat.

5. Return to **1**.
Repeat as many times as you want to.

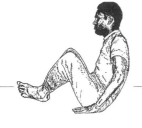

Notes for Variation 8 on the next page

If you rocked in circles when you were a child, you are likely to pick it up again quickly. Those who didn't may find they get stuck just before the **Mid-way point** and can't pull themselves up to a sitting position. If this happens, get somebody to stand behind and give you a 'shove up'. This will give you some idea of what the movement should feel like.

A friend told me his school of Martial Arts does an easier version. If you try this first, you will get a feel for it quickly and then will be able to manage the more demanding version.

Instead of catching hold of the feet, put your hands on the outside of the bent legs with the palms facing downwards, as illustrated above. Follow the same circular movements and push yourself around with your hands and elbows.

When my pupil in the picture above was a child in Tamil Nadu, India, he used to go to the beach and make circles in the sand. He used to use Malcolm Bray's version, holding on to the feet. He had competitions with his friends to see who could make the most circles in the sand. What fun!

Malcolm says he can do this on a concrete floor but you would be wise to start off on a soft surface.

Variation 8

I CALL this **Turtle Rotation**. My friend who does martial arts calls it **Diamond Rotation**, as the body is in the shape of a diamond. One of my pupil's children does it at school. They call it **Teddy Bear Roll**.

Roll over onto your right side.

Use the abdominal muscles to pull yourself up to a sitting position.

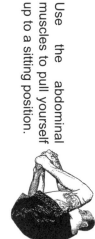
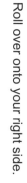
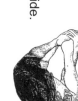

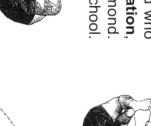

Mid-way point
The head is facing outwards again.

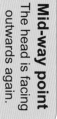
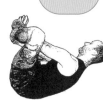

Roll over to the left.

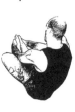
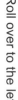

Roll over onto your back.
The head is facing inwards again.

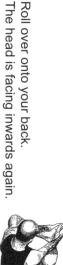

Follow the sequence in an anti-clockwise direction.

Roll over onto your back.
When you are on your back, the head is facing inwards.

Roll over to the left.

Roll over onto your back.

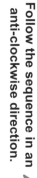

Start here
The head is facing outwards from the middle of the circle.

Go round a few times. When you are ready, change direction.

Pull up to a sitting position.

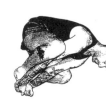

Roll over onto the right side.

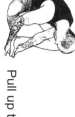

My cat, Crafty, wandered in while I was taking the photos. She came to investigate the strange things that were happening in **her** house. She looked so cute, I decided to leave her in the pictures

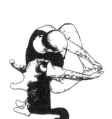
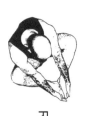

Zed and Mermaid

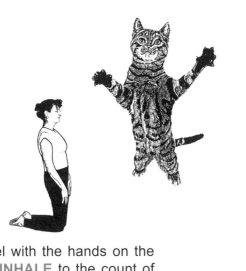

1. Kneel with the hands on the thighs. **INHALE** to the count of four.

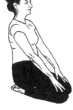

2. EXHALE to the count of eight as you lower the hips to the heels.
Repeat three times.

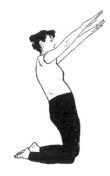

3. INHALE to the count of four as you lift the hips and raise the hands just above shoulder level.

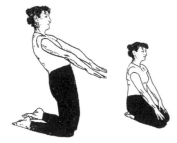

4. EXHALE to the count of eight as you lower your hands to the thighs and sink backwards onto the heels.
Repeat three times.

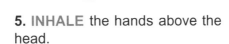

5. INHALE the hands above the head.

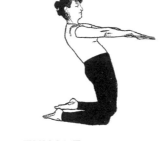

6. EXHALE as you lean backwards and lower the hands to shoulder level coming into the **Zed**.
Repeat 5 and 6, three times. The third time, hold and breathe.

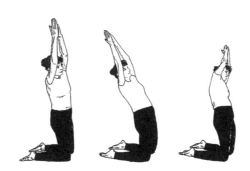

7. Return to **5** and then circle the body above the knees clockwise three times, and then anticlockwise three times.

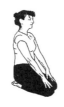

8. Return to **2**.

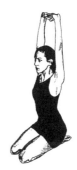

9. INHALE the hands into **Venus Lock** with the palms facing upwards. Hold for a few breaths, pushing upwards with the hands.

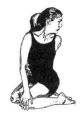

10. Let the hips fall to the right so that the feet are on the left. **EXHALE** as you lean over to the left. **INHALE** back.
Repeat three times.

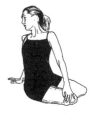

11. Place your right hand on your left knee and your left hand behind your back. Stay in the postures for a few breaths, twisting round on the exhalations.

12. Twist round the other way, with your left hand on your right knee. Place your right hand on the floor behind. You can bend the elbow to increase the stretch up the front of your body.

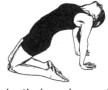

13. Place both hands on the floor behind with the fingers facing backwards. Raise the hips and hold for a few breaths in the **Backward Mermaid**. Squeeze the shoulder blades together and let the head fall back if it is comfortable.
Change sides and repeat from 9 to 13.

The Crow Sequence

IT IS easy to feel negative about the **Crow** posture. Those who find it difficult often give up, but there can be an immediate improvement after practising the preparatory postures. They help concentrate the energy in the hands and wrists. However some people find that they are too tired to do the **Crow** by the time they get to the end of the sequence. If you have weak hands and wrists avoid these postures or proceed with caution.

Some people don't like the pressure of the elbows on the legs. This prevents them from holding the posture. This can be overcome by placing a wad of firm foam in the appropriate places.

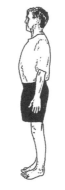
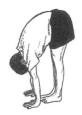

1. Stand with the feet together and the arms by your sides. **INHALE**.

2. EXHALE as you slide your hands down your legs. Bend your elbows and bring the chest towards the thighs. Hold for a few breaths in the **Standing Forward Bend.**

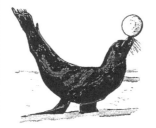

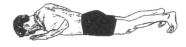

6. Lie on the floor, face downwards, with the hands under the shoulders and the elbows tucked in. Go up on your toes with the legs slightly apart.

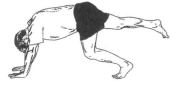
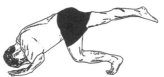

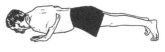

5. With the left knee still bent, lift the right leg as high as you can. Point your toes. **EXHALE** as you bend your elbows and lower the head to the floor. **INHALE** up and **EXHALE** down a few times, like a 'press up'. This is less demanding with the hands further away from the feet. If you want to make it more demanding, move the hand backwards.
Change sides and repeat.

7. INHALE as you push up on your hands and lift your body off the floor. The hips should be a little higher than the shoulders and the chin forwards. I call this the **Excruciating Posture** as most people find it demanding. Hold for as long as you comfortably can.
Lower and repeat if you want to.

Sitting Forward Bend Variation

THIS IS another of Bob Camp's contributions. My pupils find it enjoyable and beneficial. He says; ***This is intended for people like myself who have always found the forward bend difficult.*** Those who have tight muscles in the backs of their legs find this posture and the **Dog** demanding. They may find they have to bend their knees a little.

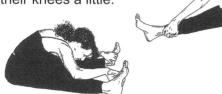
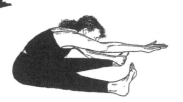
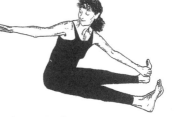

1. Sit with the legs wide and your palms wrapped around the insteps of your feet. If you cannot reach that far, wrap your palms around the inside of your lower legs, as illustrated. Keep the knees as straight as you can. Hold for a few breaths and gently ease yourself forwards on the exhalations.

2. Stretch your right hand away, in between the feet, as far forward as you can. Hold for a few breaths and push away.

3. Swing your right hand round to the right. Keep the chest high. Hold for a few breaths. You can use your left hand as a lever to help you twist round more.
Repeat **2** and **3**, three times.
Change sides and repeat.

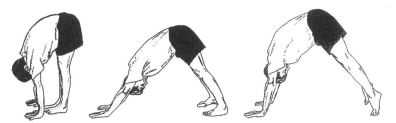 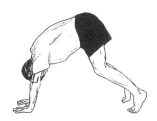

3. Place your hands on the floor and walk them forwards until you are in the **Dog** posture. Swing forwards, put your weight on your hands and go up on tiptoes. Swing backwards and forwards a few times until you feel your energy concentrated in your hands.

4. Bend the knees and repeat.

GO BACK TO PAGE 50

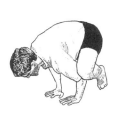 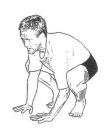 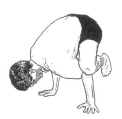

8. Squat down on all fours and go up on the toes. Make a square with your hands and feet. You may like to turn the fingers inwards. Bend your elbows and work your knees up the upper arms. When they can't go any higher, move the head and shoulders forwards. Look forwards. Don't try to lift the feet. Feel them leaving the floor as the head and shoulders move forwards. Hold for as long as you comfortably can.

9. Repeat **8**, but this time, with the feet together and the hands wider apart. It is important to look forwards.

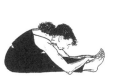 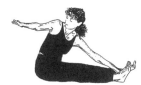

6. Now repeat the whole sequence with the feet together.

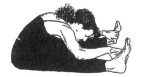 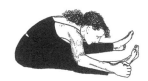

4. Return to **1**. Holding with both hands again, gently ease yourself forwards on the exhalations.

5. When you are ready, move your hands to the outside of your feet or legs. Continue to ease yourself forwards. **Caution:** Do not over stretch. I once hurt my back trying too hard in the **Sitting Forward Bend**.

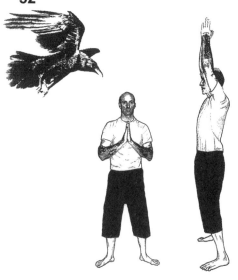

The Low Crow

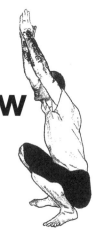

1. Stand with the feet fairly wide and the hands in **Prayer** with the thumbs crossed over. **INHALE** as you stretch your hands above your head.

2. EXHALE as you lower into a deep **Indian Squat**. Look up at your hands. Hold and breathe.

Introduction

THIS IS one of Malcolm Bray's sequences. I have presented a basic outline but, when Malcolm teaches it he varies it. Here are a few suggestions. Go from **1**, with the arms raised, to **2** at least three times. Malcolm says this is a particularly good stretch for the middle and lower back.

The **Low Crow**, **8**, can be practised after **6** by walking the feet towards the hands. This is **7** in reverse. You can go forwards a few times and repeat the **Low Crow** to work out the abdominal muscles. To conclude, proceed from **7** onwards.

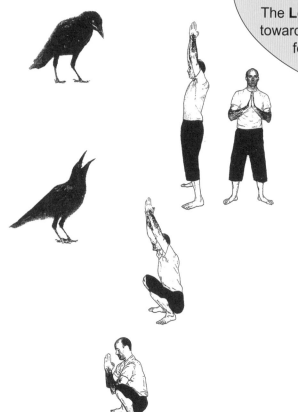

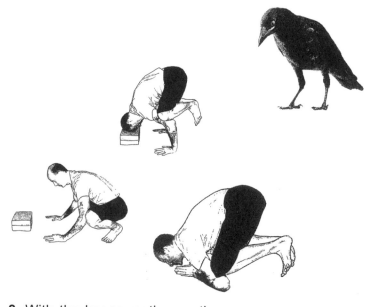

9. When you are ready, return your feet to the floor and come to a standing position, moving through **3**, **2** and **1**.

8. With the knees resting on the upper arms, move your head and shoulders forwards until the feet come off the floor. This is a **Low Crow**.
If you find this posture too demanding, try the variation illustrated above. Use blocks or firm cushions to support the head.

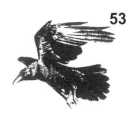

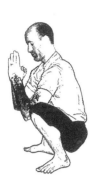

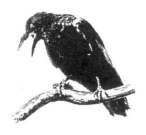

3. EXHALE the hands down bringing the elbows inside your knees.

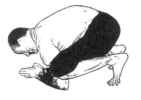

4. Go up on your toes as you lower your forearms to the floor.

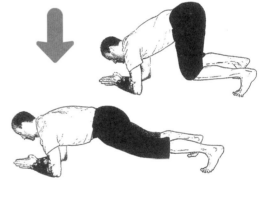

5. Walk your arms forwards until your legs are straight. This will involve some undulation of the body.

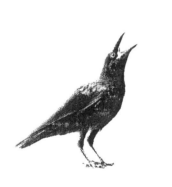

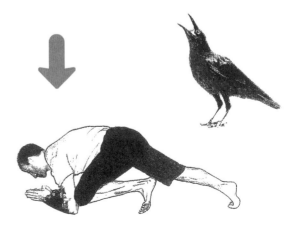

6. After you have settled in the posture, swing your left knee forwards bringing it to the outside of your elbow. Return to **5**.
Change sides and repeat.

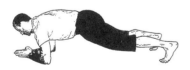

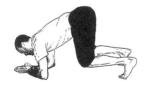

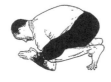

7. Walk your arms backwards returning to **4**. This is **5** in reverse.

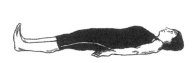

1. Lie on your back with your toes towards your head and your arms close to your sides. If you have lower back problems, bend the left knee.

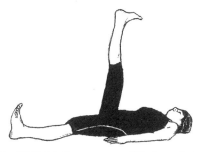

2. INHALE as you lift the right leg. **EXHALE** it down.
Repeat three times.

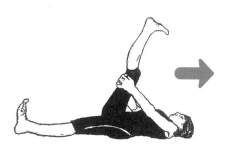

3. Catch hold of your lower thigh with both hands. Interlock the fingers and pull the leg back towards your head. Push the heel away, extending and straightening the leg.
Rotate your right foot clockwise at least three times and the same anticlockwise.

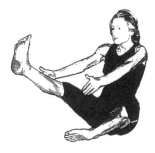

16. Remove the left hand and lift the right leg high in front. Bring your arms up to knee level with the palms facing and hold in the **Half Boat**.
Return to 11. Change sides and repeat.

Leg Raise Sequence

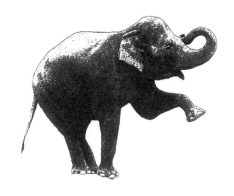

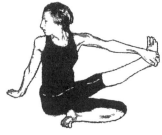

15. Lower the leg and bring it in front. Put your left hand over the top of your right foot and straighten the right leg out to the left. Place your right hand on the floor behind and twist round to the right. You can experiment with lifting the right hand if you want to.

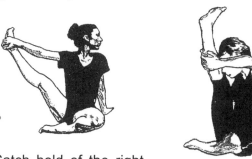

14. Catch hold of the right heel with the right hand. Place your left hand on the floor behind and twist round to the left. After a few breaths you can lift the left hand and twist round a bit more.

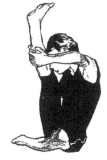

13. Lower the hands to the calf and bring the leg further back.

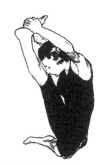

12. EXHALE as you bend your elbows and bring your head to the knee.

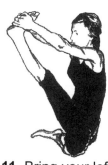

11. Bring your left heel in, close to the body. Take hold of your right foot with both hands. **INHALE** as you straighten the leg.

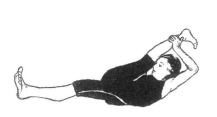

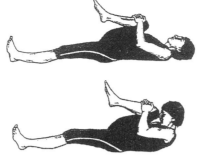

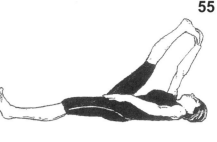

4. Move your hands up your leg. Bend the elbows and bring the head to the knee. Try to keep the right knee straight. The left heel should stay on the floor but you can soften the knee and let it bend a little.
Change sides and repeat.

5. Lower the head. Interlock your fingers on the top of the knee and hug it close to you. Push away forcefully with the left heel. **EXHALE** as you bring your head to your knee. Hold and breathe.
Return to 2. Change sides and repeat.

6. Lift your right foot and catch hold of your toes with the right hand. Place the left hand on the left thigh. **INHALE** as you straighten the right leg. If you can't straighten the leg while holding on to the toes, move the hand lower down the leg.

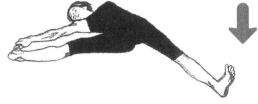

7. **INHALE** your right leg out to the side. The left hip will very probably come off the floor. Try to broaden out the hips by easing it down. You can apply gentle pressure with the left hand. Keep the left shoulder low. You may prefer to place the left hand on the floor with the palm facing downwards.

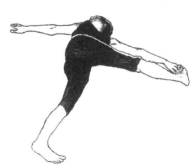

8. **INHALE** the leg up and change hands. **EXHALE** as you lower the leg to the floor on the left. Look to the right.
Return to 6. Change sides and repeat.

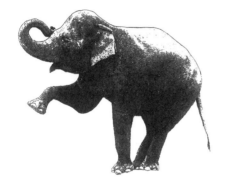

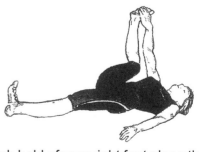

9. Catch hold of your right foot along the instep with your right hand. **INHALE** as you bring the foot and knee back and down. Hold for about 20 seconds feeling the stretch on the thigh. This is the **Stirrup Pose**. You may prefer to bend the left knee with the foot on the floor.
Change sides and repeat.

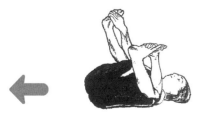

10. Catch hold of both feet and repeat in the same way. Afterwards, either rock to a sitting position holding on to the ankles, or roll over to the right and sit up.

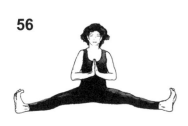

1. Sit with the legs wide and the toes back towards your head. Push the back of the knees down to the floor.
INHALE the hands into **Prayer**.

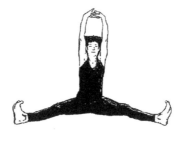

2. Interlock the fingers in **Venus Lock** with the palms facing upwards. Push away with the heels and stretch the hands over your head.

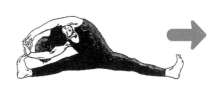

3. EXHALE the hands down to the right. Rotate your right shoulder forwards and your left shoulder backwards.
Look up to the ceiling. Feel the rotation around the waist and up the spine.
Repeat 2 and 3, three times.
Change sides and repeat.

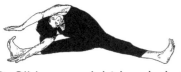
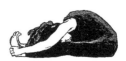

18. Slide your right hand along the floor on the inside of your leg, palm facing downwards. Lower the left arm over your head and push both hands over to the right. Rotate the left shoulder backwards. Hold and breathe, twisting round more on the exhalations.

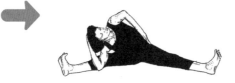

19. Bring your right elbow into the centre and lower it to the floor. Rest the hand on your head. Place the left hand on the hip and continue to twist round as before.

20. Bring the feet together. Repeat the movements of the hands with the breath as in **9**.
Repeat three times.
Hold the last stretch and lower the hands down to the feet in the **Sitting Forward Bend**.
Bend your elbows and bring your head forwards and down. For a variation you can widen the legs and catch hold of the insteps of your feet.
Return to 9. Change sides and repeat.

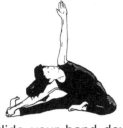

17. Slide your hand down and catch hold of your heel. **INHALE** the left hand up and rotate round, looking up at your hand.

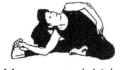

16. Move your right hand up to your toes. Adjust the angle of your hands so that you can rest your elbow on the floor or your knee. Place your left hand on your hip. Hold and breathe, twisting round to the left on the exhalations.

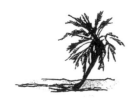

Sitting Side Stretch

 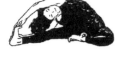

15. Slide your right hand down the outside of your foot.

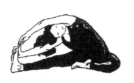

14. Maintaining the rotation, **EXHALE** as you lower your hands to the right foot. Rotate your left shoulder back and look up at the ceiling. Hold and breathe.

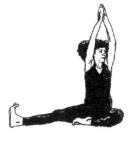

13. INHALE up. Bring your hands together above your head. Rotate round to the left from the waist upwards.

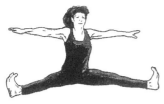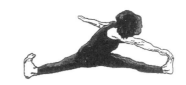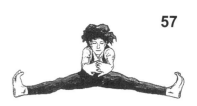

4. INHALE the hands out to the side. Lower the shoulders and push the fingers and heels away.

5. EXHALE the right hand to the left foot. Rotate your left shoulder backwards. Look at your left hand. *Change sides and repeat.*

6. INHALE back to the centre and bring the hands in to **Venus Lock**. Hold the posture and push the hands away and the head forwards and down on the exhalations.

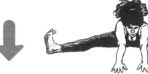

7. Lower the hands to the floor. Walk them away from you.

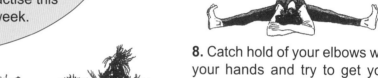

8. Catch hold of your elbows with your hands and try to get your head and elbows to the floor. If your head touches the floor, walk the elbows away from you and lower the chest to the floor.

Introduction

I CALL this sequence 'the nitty-gritty'.

We have a saying in yoga that goes;
You are as young as your spine is flexible.
This is the sequence for increasing and maintaining the flexibility of the spine and backs of the legs. If you are too busy to do any other posture work, make sure you make time to practise this one at least three times a week.

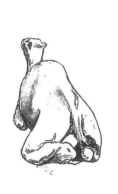

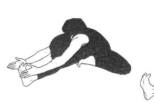

9. Place your left foot along your right thigh. **INHALE** as you bring your hands to the **Heart Centre**. **EXHALE** as you stretch the hands forward without touching your feet. *Repeat three times.* As you **INHALE** the hands back, feel yourself bringing energy back to the **Heart Centre**. **EXHALE** the hands further away each time.

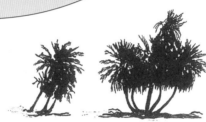

Camel Rubber Leg Contortion Posture

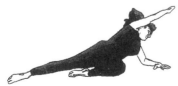

12. INHALE up and lower the left elbow down to the floor behind you. Extend your right arm over your head in the **Sciatic Stretch**. You can move your right foot back a little and point the toes. Look downwards. Hold and push away on the exhalations.

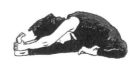

11. EXHALE them down and catch hold of the foot or lower leg.

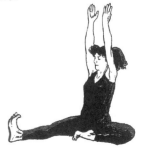

10. INHALE the hands up.

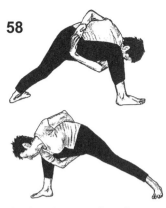

6. Slide the back of your left hand around your back and bring your right arm under the right thigh. Clasp the hands together behind your back. This is called **Binding**.

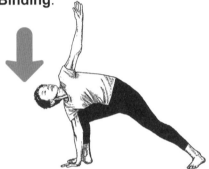

7. INHALE as you lower your right hand to the floor and twist round to the left, looking up at your left hand.

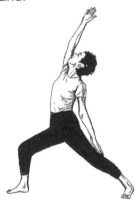

8. INHALE as you swing up and back into the **Backward Warrior**. Hold and breathe as you feel your left hand sliding down the back of your leg as your head and right arm lower to the left.

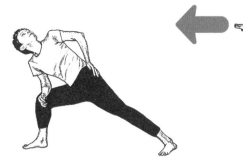

5. Place your left hand on the left hip and twist round, looking up to the left.

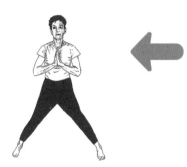

19. Return to **1**.
Change sides and repeat.

Warrior Sequence
Introduction

WHEN I was '*Googling*' for photos of Warriors to help illustrate this sequence, I observed that many were standing with their legs apart and with a bent front leg, ready to spring into action.

Yoga teachers approach this basic posture differently. Some say the front knee should be above the ankle. Others say it doesn't matter if the knee is further forwards. Some say the heels should be aligned. Others say it is best with the back foot just a few inches forwards. If you are working by yourself, keep within your comfort zone.

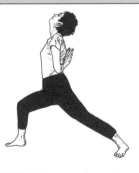

9. INHALE your head up and bring your hands behind your back in **Prayer**. EXHALE as you lean backwards.

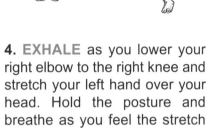

4. EXHALE as you lower your right elbow to the right knee and stretch your left hand over your head. Hold the posture and breathe as you feel the stretch along the left side of your body.

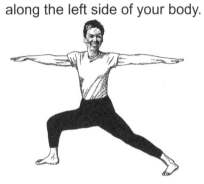

18. Lower your left foot to the floor and twist round to the left coming into the **Forward Facing Warrior**. Stretch the hands out to the sides with the palms facing downwards. Lift the chest and sink the shoulders down and back.

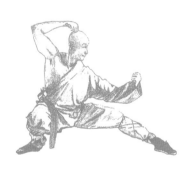

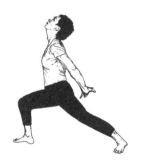

10. Bring your hands into **Venus Lock** with the palms pushing away from you. Slowly increase your backward stretch.

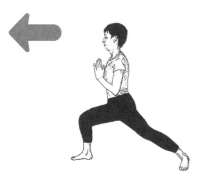

3. Bend your right knee and rotate the top part of your body over your right leg. Sink down as low as you comfortably can and roll over onto the outside of your back foot.

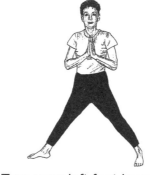

2. Turn your left foot inwards (to about a 45-degree angle) and your right foot outwards to a right angle.

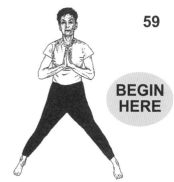

BEGIN HERE

1. Stand with the legs wide apart and the hands in **Prayer**.

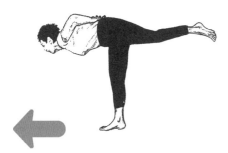

17. Place your hands in the hollow of your back with the palms facing upwards.

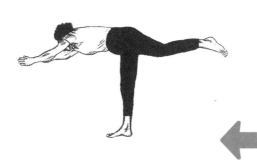

16. Separate the hands and swing forwards into **Balancing Warrior** lifting the left leg. Look up and push the hands away, with the palms facing.

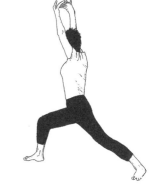

15. Twist round to the right. You will not be able to twist so far in this direction.

Breathing

Only minimal **instructions** are suggested for moving in and out of the postures. You may want to hold the postures for at least five breaths. Pace this sequence according to your level of fitness. If you are an unfit beginner, don't stay in the postures for more than a few breaths.

If you find practising the complete sequence too demanding on the front leg, you can break it up into sections. You could, for example, go as far as the **Deep Lunge (11)**, and then change sides and repeat. You would then complete the second half on both sides.

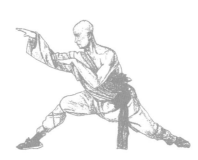

A Shaolin Warrior Monk

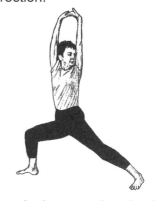

14. Interlock your hands in **Venus Lock**. Push the palms upwards. INHALE as you twist round to the left.

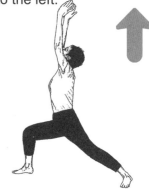

13. Swing up into the **Exultant Warrior**. Separate the hands above your head with the palms facing. Bring your chest forward and your arms back.
Looking up at your hands and leaning backwards is optional.

11. EXHALE as you swing forwards into a **Deep Lunge**.

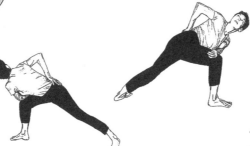

12. Twist round to the right by placing your left elbow on the right knee and your right hand on your hip.

Warrior and Starfish

THIS SEQUENCE came from a workshop given by Swami Sharadananda who teaches in and around the Basingstoke area (Southern UK). She said she *allowed it to evolve as a natural sequence from the flow of internal energy*. She has also added arrows to some of my drawings to indicate how this flow of energy can be experienced. It is a majestic sequence with large expansive movements.

Notes on the illustrations: *For the Shaolin Warrior Monks of China, their posture work and martial arts were both a spiritual discipline and a necessity. Monasteries had to be protected and they were called upon to fight battles against pirates and other disruptive elements. To see them in action, go to* YouTube, Shaolin Monks, Empty Mind. *For more information, visit* Wikipedia.

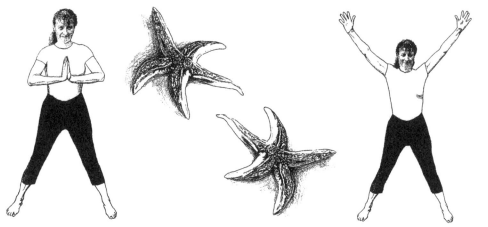

1. Stand with the feet wide apart and the hands in **Prayer**.

2. **INHALE** the hands up into **Starfish** with the fingers spread out and the palms facing forwards.

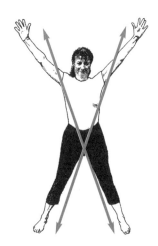

10. When you are ready, turn the feet to face forwards and return to the **Starfish**. *Change sides and repeat.*

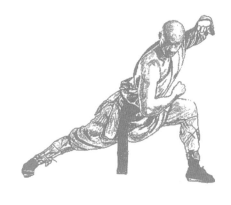

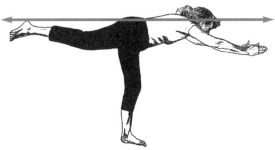

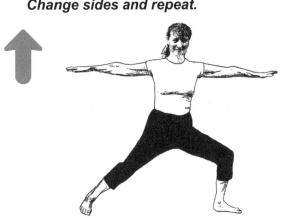

9. Lower your right leg to the floor and swing round into **Forward Facing Warrior**.

8. Mentally prepare to come into the **Balancing Warrior** or **Warrior 3**. Shift your weight onto your left leg. Soften the knee as you lift your right leg and swing your hands forwards with the palms facing each other.
Look up and straighten the left leg.
Hold for a few breaths.

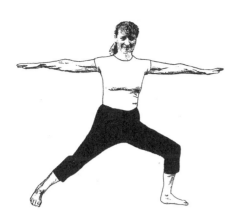

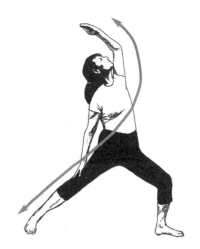

3. Turn your right foot inwards and your left foot outwards. As you **EXHALE**, bend your left knee and bring your hands out to the sides with the palms facing downwards.

Hold for a few breaths, rolling onto the outside of your back foot.

Lift the chest and drop the shoulders down and back. Push away with your fingers.

This is **Forward Facing Warrior** or **Warrior 2**.

4. Place your right hand on the back of your right leg and lean backwards, coming into the **Backward Warrior**. Look up at your left hand and sink down as low as you can. Hold for a few breaths, gradually sliding your right hand down the back of your leg.

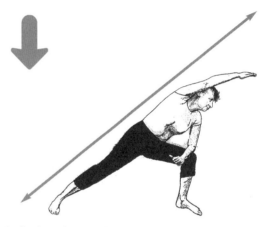

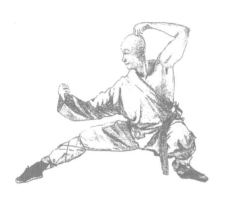

5. Swing forwards, bringing your left elbow onto your left knee. Stretch your right hand over your head. Continue to roll over onto the outside of your back foot and stretch all the way up the right side of your body.

Hold for a few breaths.

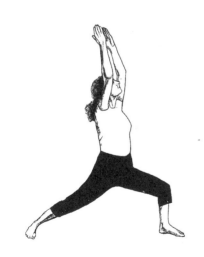

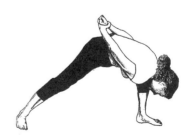

7. INHALE up into the **Warrior or Warrior 1**. Adjust your feet if necessary. The hands are separate with the palms facing. Bring the arms back and the chest forwards. Look up at your hands. Straighten the elbows and push away with your fingers. Hold for a few breaths.

6. INHALE as you bring your hands into **Venus Lock** behind your back. Push the palms away from you. **EXHALE** as you lower your head down the inside of your left leg. Move the hands upwards and the head as low as you can in a **Deep Lunge**.

Toe Pull Sequence

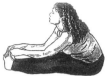

1. Sit with the legs forwards and the toes back towards the head. Catch hold of the big toes or the lower legs if you can't stretch that far. Bend the elbows and pull the chest forwards and up. Lower the shoulders and look up. The back should be straight not curved. Hold for a few breaths feeling the stretch on the back of the legs.

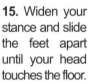

15. Widen your stance and slide the feet apart until your head touches the floor. *Proceed with caution.* If you are not able to stretch that far, go as far down as you safely can. If necessary, put your hands on the floor. Come out of the posture carefully. ***You may repeat the sequence as many times as you want to.***

14. INHALE as you move the hips back a little and look up. Feel the weight on your heels and pull the chest into the thighs.

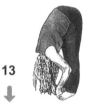
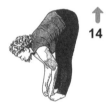

13. Lower your feet to the floor. **INHALE** as you slowly come to a standing position. **EXHALE** as you lower your head and catch hold of the big toes. Bend the elbows and bring the head down and in. Hold for a few breaths, feeling the stretch on the back of the legs.

12. Return to **3**.

11. Return to **4**.

10. Go straight into **5**.

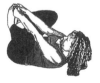

9. Bend the knees bringing the feet together in the middle. Lift the head a little. You may prefer to catch hold of the ankles at this point. Rock to an upright position without letting the feet touch the floor in front. This may take a bit of practise.

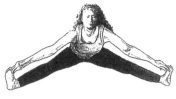
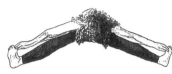

2. Widen the legs and catch hold of the big toes. **INHALE** with the head up and **EXHALE** as you lower it down. ***Repeat three times.***

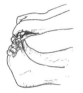

IF YOU can't reach your big toes, hold on to your ankles or lower legs.

You may hold the big toes by wrapping the first finger around and pressing the sides with the thumbs or with the first two fingers on the back of the toe and the thumb on the nail.

Breathing advice is difficult in this sequence as the breath will 'have a mind of its own' when moving between the postures. Rather be an observer than a controller. Hold the postures for as long as you want to.

Caution

Make sure there are no obstructing objects behind you before you start this sequence as you will be rocking backwards.

Make sure the spine is well cushioned with layers of mats and blankets.

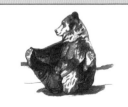
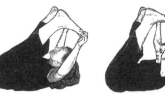

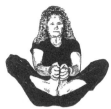

3. Sit up and bring your feet together. Catch hold of the toes with each hand and lift the feet as high and as close to the body as you can. Drop the shoulders and stretch the top of your head towards the ceiling. Hold for a few breaths in the **Balancing Cobbler**.

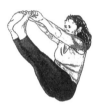

4. INHALE as you straighten the legs towards the ceiling. You can bend them if necessary. Hold and breathe. Keep the head forwards so that you don't roll backwards.

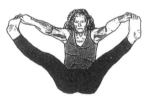

5. INHALE as you swing your legs out to the sides, coming into the **Wide Sitting Balance**.

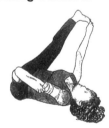

6. Allow yourself to roll backwards into the **Partridge**. Hold and breathe.

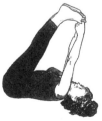

7. When you are ready bring the legs together, coming into the **Supine Toe Pull**.

8. Lift your head and shoulders and rock backwards and forwards. The legs can be wide or together. Try to get your feet to the floor behind you.

Cobbler and Frog

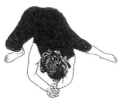

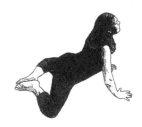

9. Come up onto the forearms into **Frog in Sphinx**. Lower the chin forwards. The elbows can go out to the sides. Sink the spine and chest downwards. The spine is in a strong **Dog Tilt** *(see the **Cat Sequence** page 32)* for **9**, **10** and **11**.

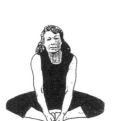

1. Sit with the soles of the feet together and catch hold of your toes. Butterfly the knees down to the floor in the **Cobbler**.

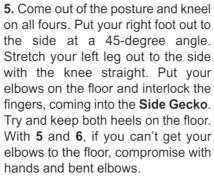

5. Come out of the posture and kneel on all fours. Put your right foot out to the side at a 45-degree angle. Stretch your left leg out to the side with the knee straight. Put your elbows on the floor and interlock the fingers, coming into the **Side Gecko**. Try and keep both heels on the floor. With **5** and **6**, if you can't get your elbows to the floor, compromise with hands and bent elbows.

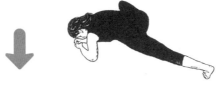

6. Move your left leg back and go up on the toes. The hands and right foot return to where they were in **5**. This is the **Gecko**. Hold for a few breaths pushing your right thigh and knee out to the side.
Change sides and repeat 5 and 6.

10. Keeping the feet and knees as they are, bring the hands back and straighten the arms, lifting the chest up. Swing the hips forwards and look up. Widen the knees a little, stretching the inner thighs, in the **Upward Frog**.

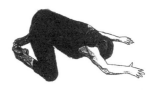

11. Move the feet out to the sides in the **Wide Upward Frog**.

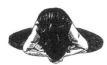

2. INHALE with the head up and EXHALE as you lower your head to your toes. ***Repeat three times.***

3. Slide your feet forwards and put your hands under your feet. Hold for a few breaths, slowly lowering your head to your feet.

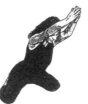

7. Come out of the posture. Sit with the knees wide and the hips resting on the feet with the big toes touching. INHALE the hands up in **Prayer**. Tilt the abdomen forwards. Lean forwards and push away with the hands. This is the **Leaping Frog**.

12. Either keep the feet wide or bring them back together. Swing the hips back and rest the forehead on the floor. Sink the chest down towards the floor and rest in the **Wide Lizard**.

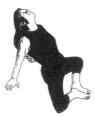

4. Place your hands behind you on the floor with the fingers turned out to the sides. Lift the buttocks off the floor. Expand the chest forwards and squeeze the shoulder blades together.
The head can drop back if it is comfortable. Hold for a few breaths, pushing the knees downwards in the **Backward Cobbler**.

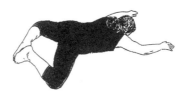

8. Keeping the feet and knees as they are, lower the chest down to the floor, coming into the **Frog**. Stretch out the arms and fingers wide in front. The chin is forwards.

13. Return to **1**, **2** and **3**. You may find your flexibility has increased a little.

64

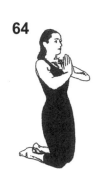

1. Kneel with the hands in **Prayer**.

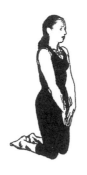

2. Lower your hands to the left thigh.

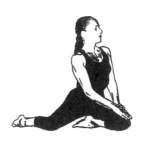

3. Bring your left knee forwards and slide the right foot backwards. Your right knee should be behind the left foot.

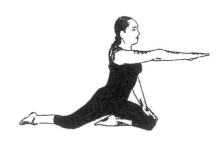

4. INHALE the right hand forwards.

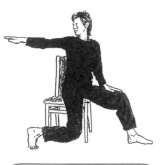

If you have bad knees, you can do this sequence sitting on the corner of a chair.

Dove Sequence

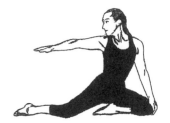

5. EXHALE the hand back and look over your right shoulder, coming into the **Dove**. **INHALE** the left hand lower down the knee and sink down as low as you can.

11. Return to **1** (above). *Change sides and repeat.*

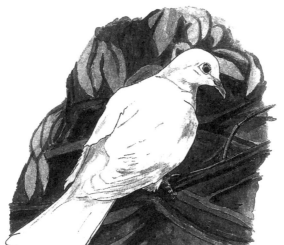
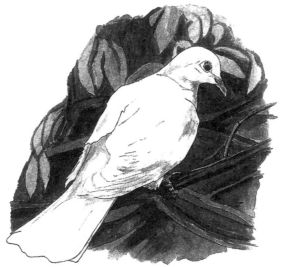

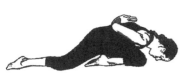

10. EXHALE the head down, coming into the **Forward Dove**.

6. Lower your hand to the back of your knee. **EXHALE** as you twist round more and look at your right hand.

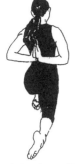

9. Lower the right leg. Bring your hands behind your back in **Prayer**, or catch hold of the elbows. Lean backwards in the **Backward Dove**.

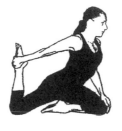

7. Bring your right hand behind your back and catch hold of the left elbow. Hold and twist round more on the exhalations in the **Twisting Dove**.

8. Bend the right knee, and catch hold of your foot with the right hand. Place the left hand on the knee or the floor.

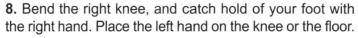

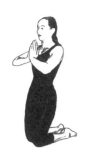

1. Kneel with the hands in **Prayer**.

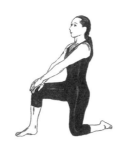

2. INHALE the right foot forward and place the hands on your knee.

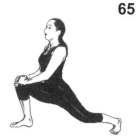

3. EXHALE as you lift the left knee off the floor and go up on your toes.

The Equestrian Twist Sequence

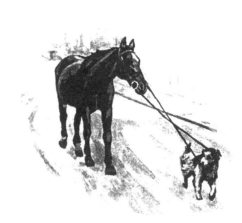

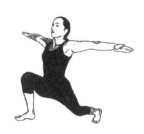

4. INHALE the hands into **Prayer** above your head.

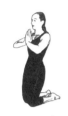

13. Return to **1**.
Change sides and repeat.

5. EXHALE the hands down. INHALE as you stretch the hands out to the sides.

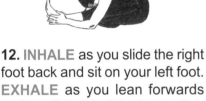

12. INHALE as you slide the right foot back and sit on your left foot. EXHALE as you lean forwards and catch hold of the leg as low down as you can. Lower your head to your knee.

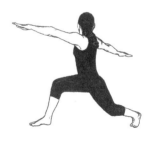

6. EXHALE as you twist to the right.

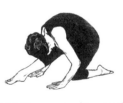

11. INHALE as you lower the left knee to the floor and straighten the right leg. EXHALE as you lower the head to the knee.

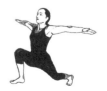

7. INHALE back to **5**.

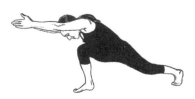

10. EXHALE the hands forwards into **Prayer** and straighten the left leg.

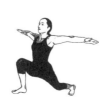

9. INHALE back to **5**.　　**8.** EXHALE round to the left.

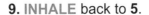

The Hip Swing Sequence

AS THE instructions are the same for every posture in this sequence, I am giving general guidelines at the beginning.

INHALE before you prepare to swing the hips over and **EXHALE** as you swing them over.
Hold each posture for at least four breaths and keep pushing over to the side.
Keep both shoulders on the floor unless instructed otherwise.
Both hips come off the floor and you will be lying on your side.
Change sides and repeat each posture before moving on to the next.

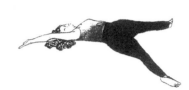

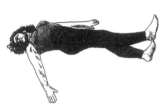

1. Lie on your back. Put your right foot on top of your left foot. The heel can go between the big toe and the second toe. Look to the right and swing the hips and feet over to the left into the **Flat Twist**.
Follow the instructions above.

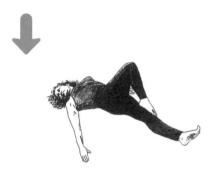

2. Wrap your right foot around your left knee. Look to the right and swing the hips over to the left.

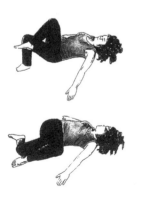

3. Bend your left knee. Keep your foot on the floor and place your right foot on the outside of your left knee. Look to the right and swing your hips and knees over to the left. Try to place the right foot on the floor.

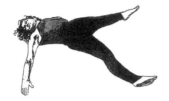

4. With both legs straight, lift your right leg. Look to the right and swing your right leg over to the left.

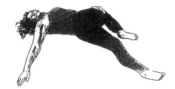

5. Bend your right knee. Lift the foot. Place your left hand on your right knee. Look to the right and pull the knee over to the left. You can put a little pressure on the knee with the left hand.
After a few breaths you can let your right shoulder come off the floor and lower your right knee down to the floor. If your neck feels uncomfortable you can look up to the ceiling.

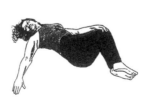

6. Bend both knees and bring them up to the chest. Put your left hand on the outside of your right knee. Pull the knees over to the left. You can put a little pressure on the top knee with the left hand.

7. With both legs straight, move the feet to the right. Lift the right leg and swing it over to the left. The buttocks will come off the floor. Lower the right big toe to the floor.
Swing your right arm backwards and look back at your hand. Stretch all the way along the right side of the body from the toes to the fingers.

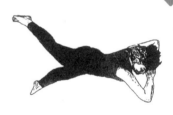

8. Roll over onto the abdomen. Put one hand on top of the other. Rest your left ear on your hands, looking to the right.
Lift your right leg as high as you can and swing it round over the top of your left leg.

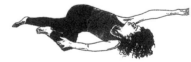

9. Slide your right knee up the side of your body, as high as it will go. Put your left hand under the chest and place it on top of your right knee. Swing the right arm back and look up at your hand.
You will find the head sometimes rests on the floor, and doesn't at other times.

The Shoulder Stand Sequence

PLEASE READ the 'Cautions and Health Issues' section on page 8 and the important caution box on page 69 before you attempt this sequence.

If you are overweight, you are likely to find breathing difficult in the **Shoulder Stand (3)** and the **Inverted Dragon Fly (17)**. You are likely to find the angle of the body in the **Inverted Posture (2)** more comfortable.

Some people find placing a folded blanket about 1½ inches (4 cm) thick under the shoulders helps to ease the pressure on the neck.

The most commonly recommended time to stay in the **Shoulder Stand** is up to three minutes. Some teachers say that to stay in it longer is like over-watering plants.

The **Shoulder Stand** is traditionally followed by the **Bridge** or the **Fish**. They are considered counter postures.

Alternative Endings

1   If you have long legs, you are likely to find going straight from the **Shoulder Stand** to the **Bridge** an enjoyable way to end this sequence. Those with short legs may struggle. If you are a beginner and working by yourself, do not attempt this unless you feel very confident.

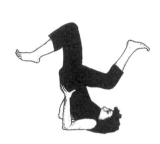

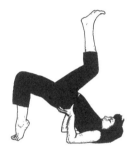

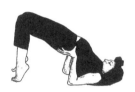

1. Make a firm support for your back with your hands.
Lower one knee down to your head to steady the ascent. Bend the other knee.

2. Slowly lower the front leg until the toes touch the floor.

3. Lower the other leg coming into the **High Bridge**. When you are ready, lower the heels to the floor.

2   If you can already do the **Lotus** posture, you will find approaching it from the **Shoulder Stand** a good way to get into the posture.

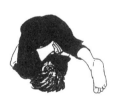

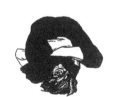

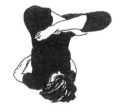

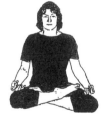

1. Bring the knees down behind you, towards the floor, catch hold of your preferred foot with the opposite hand and bring it across the opposite thigh. Return the hand to your back.

2. Repeat with the other hand and foot.

3. With both hands on your back, raise the legs in the **Lotus** posture.

4. Place the hands on the floor, with your palms downwards. Press on the palms as you slowly lower forwards into a sitting position.
Bring your hands into **Chin Mudra**, with the thumbs and first fingers forming a circle, and place the back of your hands on your knees.

The Shoulder Stand and Figures of Eight

You can make figures of eight, **8**, with your legs and feet while holding the **Shoulder Stand**. First work from side to side. Make a small circle with one foot and another with the other foot. Change direction when you are ready. Then you can try with the feet together. You can also make an **8** with the feet together, going forwards and backwards. Make a small circle in front and a much larger one behind.

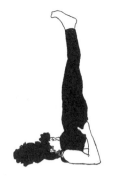

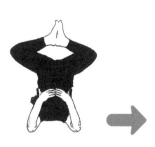

1. Lie on your back with your arms close to your sides, palms downwards.

2. **INHALE** up into the **Inverted Posture**. Place your hands on your back with the thumbs on the outside and the fingers spread out. The legs slope backwards.

3. **INHALE** the feet towards the ceiling and move the hips towards your head. Hold and breathe in the **Shoulder Stand**.

4. **EXHALE** the soles of the feet together, coming into the **Closed Scissors**.

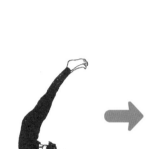

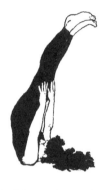

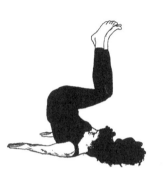

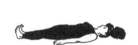

21. Return to **19**.

22. Very slowly bring your hands, one at a time, onto the thighs. This is the **Candle**.

23. Bring your hands to the floor in front. Press down with the palms and, vertebra by vertebra (segments of the spine), slowly lower your body to the floor. The legs can be straight or bent.

24. Return **1**.

The Shoulder Stand Sequence

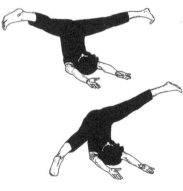

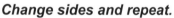

20. Repeat **6** and **8** with the arms on the floor.
Change sides and repeat.

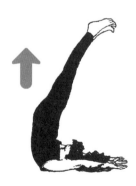

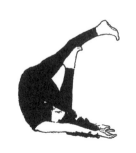

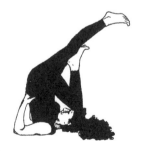

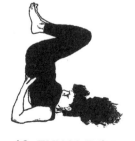

19. **INHALE** both feet up to the ceiling. This is the **Full Shoulder Stand**.

18. When you are ready, bring your hands behind your head.

17. Move your right knee onto your forehead. Bring your left leg a little into the centre and place your right foot on your left knee. Hold and breathe in the **Inverted Dragon Fly**.
Change sides and repeat.

16. **EXHALE** the knees together.

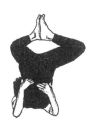 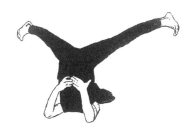 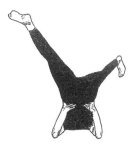 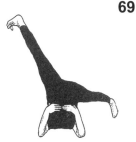

5. **INHALE** as you move the right knee forwards and the left knee back. **EXHALE** in the opposite direction.
This is the **Corkscrew**.

6. **INHALE** the feet out to the sides into the **Wide Scissors**. Flex and point the feet a few times to extend the stretch.

7. Corkscrew in the **Open Scissors**.

8. Lower your right foot to the floor to the side. Push away with the left foot. Hold and breathe.
Change sides and repeat.

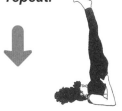

9. **INHALE** back to the **Shoulder Stand**.

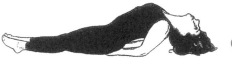 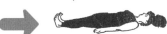

25. Place your arms under the body with the hands under the hips with the palms facing downwards. Straighten the elbows and move the hands towards the feet. **INHALE** as you lift the head and shoulders and look at your feet. Walk your elbows closer together. Arch the spine and chest forwards and upwards. **EXHALE** as you lower your head to the floor, coming into the **Fish**. Take three long slow deep breaths. Arch the back a little more with each breath.

26. To return to **1**, **INHALE** as you lift the head and tuck in the chin. **EXHALE** as you lower the head and shoulders to the floor.

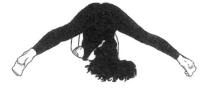

10. **EXHALE** the feet down to the floor, wide apart, coming into the **Wide Plough**.

CAUTION

ALWAYS keep facing directly upwards when in Shoulderstand or Plough. **NEVER** turn your head or even try to look to one side, when in this or similar postures.

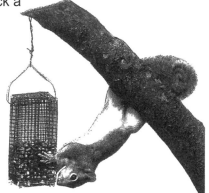

11. **INHALE** the hands up into **Prayer**.

12. **EXHALE** the hands down and catch hold of your feet.

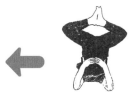 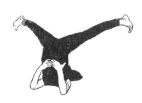 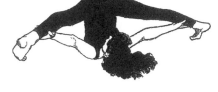

15. Return to **4**.

14. Place your hands on your back again and return to **6**.

13. **INHALE** the legs a short distance off the floor and place your hands on the lower legs. Rest in the **Wide Pose of Tranquillity**.

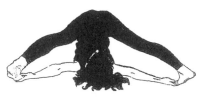

The Lion's Roar

A LION'S roar is a very loud, powerful noise; it can be heard for miles around. When you are living in lion territory the noise dominates the area at certain times of the day[1]. The sound becomes part of your daily experience. It sinks into the subconscious mind and manifests in all sorts of interesting ways[2].

You will need to practise the different ways of doing the **Lion's Roar** before you try out the sequence. You can make a **throat roar** (a sensation in the throat) or a **nose roar** (the sensation is in the top of the mouth, against the hard palate and back of the nose). The sound should never be strained. If you have a cold or sore throat, make a very quiet roar.

In a throat roar there will be diaphragm awareness and it will be difficult to flare the nostrils. In a nose roar it will be easier to flare the nostrils and you will be aware of the ribs descending during the exhalation.

A lion's roar is not always aggressive. It can be playful, experimental, communicative or an expression of pleasure. It can be in **Sympathetic** or **Parasympathetic** mode.

1. *I discovered this magic while staying at the Sivananda Ashram at Neyyar Dam, Kerala, S. India. The lions lived in the Nature Reserve across the valley.*
2. *A Google search reveals a mountain of creative resonance coming from the Lion's Roar, e.g.* The Lion's Roar: Two Discourses of the Buddha. www.lionsroar.name/lions-roar-sutra.html

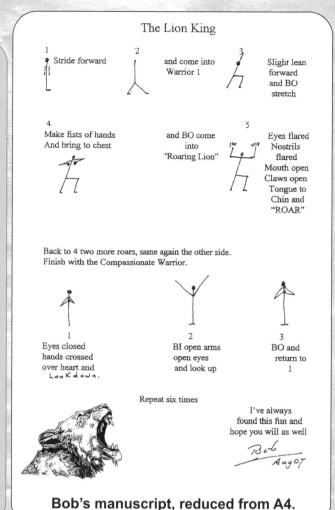

The Lion King

1 Stride forward
2 and come into Warrior 1
3 Slight lean forward and BO stretch
4 Make fists of hands And bring to chest
5 and BO come into "Roaring Lion"
Eyes flared Nostrils flared Mouth open Claws open Tongue to Chin and "ROAR"

Back to 4 two more roars, same again the other side. Finish with the Compassionate Warrior.

1 Eyes closed hands crossed over heart and Look down.
2 BI open arms open eyes and look up
3 BO and return to 1

Repeat six times

I've always found this fun and hope you will as well

Bob
Aug 07

Bob's manuscript, reduced from A4.

How the 'Lion's Roar Sequence' evolved

In August 2007, after reading *Yoga Sequences, Book 2*, Bob Camp, an experienced yoga teacher from Norfolk, very kindly sent me his 'Lion King' sequence. I have changed the name for copyright reasons. My pupils enjoyed doing it and it evolved.

Bob developed an interest in WW1 whilst visiting the graves of his relatives. He visited the Western Front several times, found the 'Brooding Warrior' very moving, and it is on this that he has based the **Compassionate Warrior**. The 'Brooding Warrior' is a memorial for the Canadian dead in Belgium. It is a solid granite column, carved to form the bowed head and shoulders of a Canadian soldier, his hands resting on the reversed rifle. He says:

The reversed rifle is standard army drill but instead of the hands crossed over the rifle butt, for the Compassionate Warrior, I show them crossed over the heart.

A friend who practises Martial Arts told me that there is a 'Lion's Roar Sequence' in that discipline. It also uses a Warrior-type posture and includes twists. This gave me the idea for twisting while roaring.

Bob's suggestion of the flared nostrils during the **Lion's Roar** made me think of a horse flaring its nostrils when it is frightened and angry. This made me think of Sophie Gabriel's idea of **Nose and Throat Breathing** in her book *Breath for Life* (see section on **Nose and Throat Breathing**). With so many sources connecting **Ujjayi** to the **Parasympathetic Nervous System**, I started to connect **Nose Breathing** to the **Sympathetic Nervous System**. I found a few examples to support the connection.

I had already started to use **Ujjayi** in the **Compassionate Warrior** so the idea of changing emotions and nervous systems during the sequences was born.

Finally, I remembered the **Fierce Pose**, and it fitted in perfectly at the end of **Version 2**.

Mastering the Lion's Roar

YOU CAN practise **1** and **2** in any position that allows you to move the top part of the body freely. **1** is a **Throat Roar** and **2** is a **Nose Roar**. If you have practised **Nose and Throat Breathing** sufficiently you will be able to differentiate between both. If you haven't, just simplify the instructions and imitate the illustrations.

1

a. Sit with your hands at the top of the thighs with the fingers spread out. Take a deep **Ujjayi** breath.

b. **EXHALE** as you slide the hands down the thighs to the knees and stretch the fingers out as wide as you can. Stick out your tongue. Tuck in the chin but keep the back of the neck long and in line with the spine. Try not to let the neck drop forwards. Look up into the head, far enough to see black at the top of your vision. Imitate a **Lion's Roar**.

This is not an angry roar. This is the roar of a happy, contented lion. Imagine you are roaring at a full moon and the stars. *Repeat a few times.*

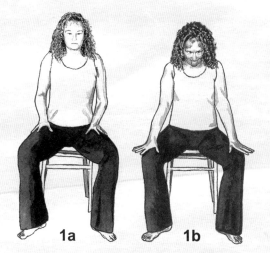

1a   1b

2

This is the way you will roar in the **Lion's Roar Sequence**. To allow a change of emotion during the sequence we will keep the roar in **Sympathetic** mode. Imagine that your survival is being threatened and you are defending yourself. Feel fierce and angry.

a. **INHALE** with a nose breath. Feel the sides of the nose being sucked together and the ribs lifting. Clench your fists and bring them on either side of the upper chest.

b. **EXHALE** with your **Lion's Roar**. Feel angry and defend your territory. Open the mouth wide and stick out your tongue. Keep your chin in line with the floor. Feel the emphasis on the top part of the mouth and back of the nose and flare your nostrils. Bring your hands up and use your fingers to mimic a lion's claws. *Repeat a few times.*

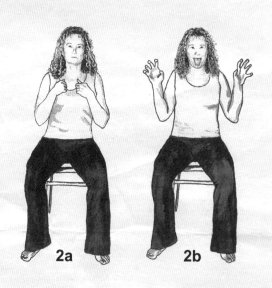

2a   2b

3

1 and **2** are a simplified version of the first technique for the **Lion's Pose** described in the *Hatha Yoga Pradipika (Bihar version)*. **3** is the second technique from the same section of the book.

a. Place the hands on the ground with the fingers turned towards the thighs. In this position there is pressure on the heels of the hands.

b. **INHALE** deeply through the nose. Tuck in the chin and feel the rib-cage expanding.

c. Raise the chin 2 or 3 inches, look up into the top of the head and protrude the tongue as far as is comfortable. **EXHALE** with a **Lion's Roar**.

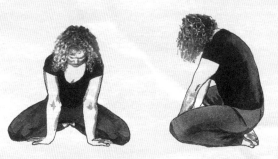

3a   3b

Swami Muktibodhana's commentary says:
This is particularly good for toning the throat and eradicating stammering. It also helps to externalize introverted people. This asana is more effective when performed outside in front of the rising sun.

With version **3**, you can experiment with a **Throat Roar** and a happy mood and a **Nose Roar** and an angry mood (as described in versions **1** and **2**).

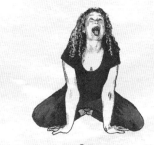

3c

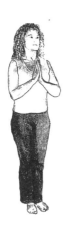

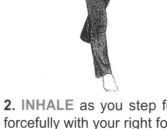

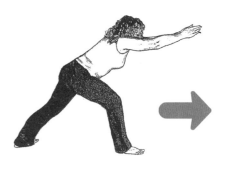

1. Stand at the back of your mat with the feet together and the hands in **Prayer** at the **Heart Centre**.

2. INHALE as you step forward forcefully with your right foot.

3. EXHALE as you bend the right knee and extend the hands forward, coming into the **Slanting Warrior**.

15. Return to **1** (see above). *Change sides and repeat.*

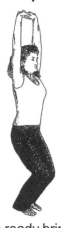

14. When you are ready bring the feet together, bend your knees and interlock the hands above your head in **Venus Lock**. Bring your chest forwards and your arms back. This is **Fierce Pose**. Return to **Nose Breathing**. Feel defensive and angry, with fierce eyes and flared nostrils.

Lion's Roar Sequence

THIS SEQUENCE offers a rare opportunity to express acceptable anger. This is therapeutic, especially when practised in groups. It is also rare to find a range of emotion in a yoga sequence.

Here is a delightful account of a young lion learning to roar from *Menagerie Manor* by Gerald Durrell (published by Summersdale. ISBN 978-1840245936).

Another newcomer was our lion, which went under the name of Leo. He was one of the famous Dublin Zoo lions (Dublin has a successful lion-breeding program), and was probably about the 50th generation born in captivity. I was glad to see, when his mane started to develop, that he was going to be a blonde lion, for, in my experience, the lions with blonde manes, as opposed to dark ones, always have nice, if slightly imbecile characters. This theory has been amply borne out by Leo's behaviour.
In his second year, Leo decided, after mature reflection, that it was a lion's duty to roar. He was not awfully sure how to go about it, so he would retire to quiet corners of his cage and practise very softly to himself, for he was rather shy of his new accomplishment and would stop immediately and pretend it was nothing to do with him if you came in view. When he was satisfied that the timbre was right and his breath control perfect, he treated us to his first concert. It was a wonderful moonlit night when he started, and we were all delighted that Leo was, at last, a proper lion.

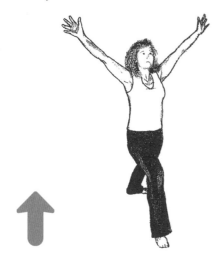

13. INHALE as you lift your arms wide and look up.

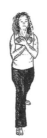

12. After returning to the centre, bend the right knee. Push up on your right foot and return to **9**.

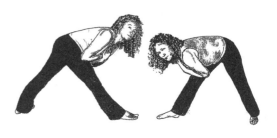

11. Lion looks up to the left. EXHALE as you twist round to the left. INHALE back to the centre. Change sides for **Lion looks up to the right**.

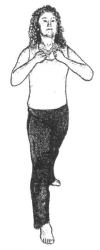

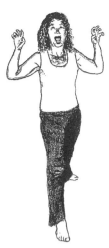

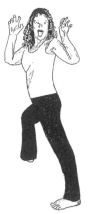

4. INHALE as you clench your fists, bring your head up and place your hands on either side of the upper chest. The front knee remains bent.

5. EXHALE into the **Lion's Roar**. This is the defensive roar, as described in the previous section.

6. The lion hears a noise behind him to the left. He twists round to the left and **Roars** at a wild boar coming out of the bushes.

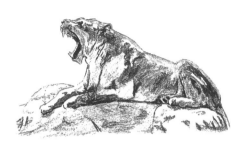

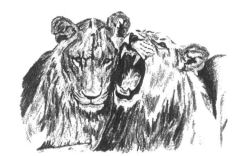

7. Return to **4** and **Roar** again.

The trouble was that Leo was so proud of his accomplishment that, from that day onwards, he could not wait until nightfall to give us the benefit of his vocal chords. He started roaring earlier and earlier each evening, and would keep it up all night, with five-minute intervals for meditation in between each roar. Sometimes, when he was in particularly good voice, you could imagine that he was sitting at the end of your bed, serenading you.

We found that if we opened the bedroom window and shouted, 'Leo, shut up', this had the effect of silencing him for half an hour, but then he would decide that you had not really meant it and would start all over again.

Later, however, Leo learnt to roar with a certain amount of discretion, but, even so, there were nights - especially during full moon - when the only thing to do was pull a pillow over your head and curse the day you ever decided you wanted a zoo.

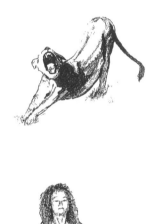

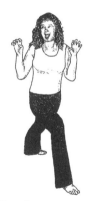

8. The lion hears a noise behind him to the right. He twists round to the right and **Roars** at an approaching elephant.

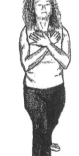

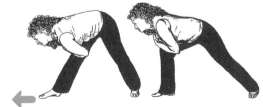

10. When you are ready, EXHALE as you lower the chest down to the thigh. INHALE as you straighten the right leg.

9. The wild boar and elephant run away and the lion has a change of mood. Cross the hands over on **Heart Centre** and look downwards in the **Compassionate Warrior**. You may close your eyes. Change to **Throat Breathing (Ujjayi)**. The lion is now passive and contented. Stay here until you feel peaceful.

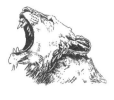

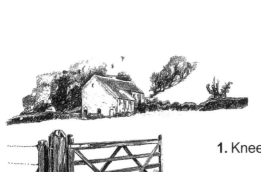

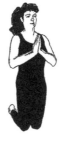

1. Kneel with the hands in **Prayer**.

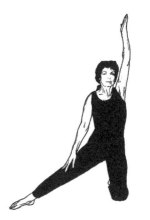

2. Stretch your right leg out to the side and place your right hand on your right knee. INHALE as you raise your left hand.

The Gate Sequence

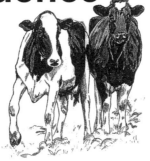

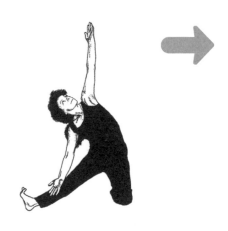

11. Return your knee to the floor and conclude with a slightly different version of **The Gate** posture.
Come up onto your right heel and place the back of your hand on your leg. INHALE your left hand up. Look up at the hand.

10. Keep your right hand on your leg. INHALE as you lift your left hand. Look up at your hand. You can stretch it away to the left.

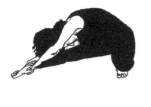

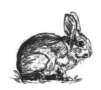

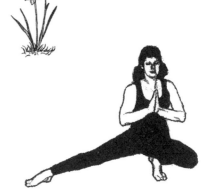

9. For the next two postures imagine that your right big toe is super-glued to the floor. Rotate over your right leg and EXHALE as you slide your hands down your leg and lower your head. You can place a hand on the floor if necessary. Hold and breathe.

8. INHALE up. Go up on your left toes, with the bent knee rotating out to the side. Bring your hands into **Prayer**. Hold and breathe in the **Balancing Gate**.

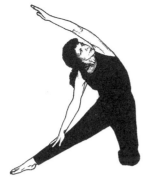
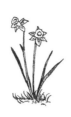
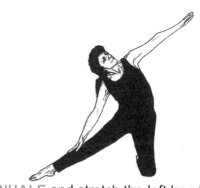

3. EXHALE as you lower down to the right. Slide the palm of your hand down your leg. This is the **Gate** posture. Look up or down but keep the left shoulder back.
Either hold for a few breaths *or* repeat three times, INHALING up and EXHALING down.

4. INHALE and stretch the left hand out to the side. Hold for a few breaths stretching the hands away from each other.

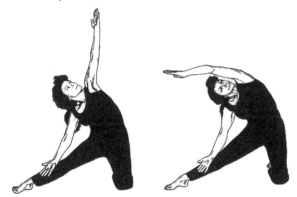

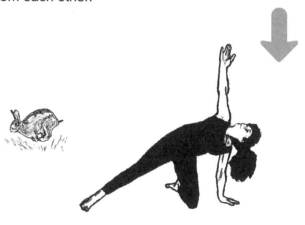

12. Lower your toes to the floor. Keep the left shoulder back as you lower your hand over your head. Hold for a few breaths, slowly increasing the stretch and feeling the increased stretch on the back of your right leg.

5. EXHALE your left hand down to the floor at the side. Lift your right hand and look up at it. Hold for a few breaths in the **Open Gate**. Stretch your right hand and toes away from each other.

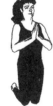

13. Return to **1**.
Change sides and repeat.

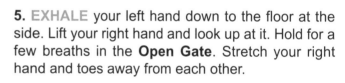

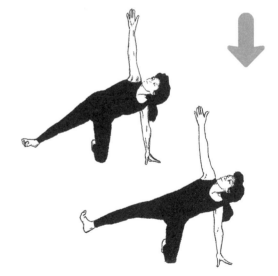

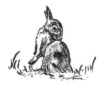

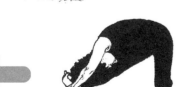

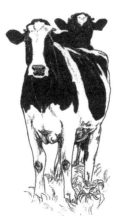
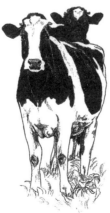

7. When you are ready, INHALE up and rotate over your right leg. EXHALE as you slide your hands down your leg and bring your head to your knee. Hold for a few breaths in the **Closed Gate**.

6. Lift your right foot a comfortable distance off the floor. Imitate a swinging gate. Bring the toes towards the head and swing the leg from side to side or up and down. You can experiment with wide and narrow swings.

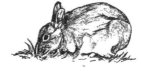

Caution. If you have had a hip replacement, you should avoid the **Swinging Gate**.

Spider in a Tree

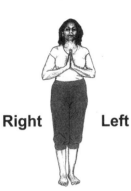

Right   **Left**

1. Stand at the right side of your mat with the feet together and the hands in **Prayer**.

Introduction

NUMBERS 4, **5** and **11 - 18** are side views. You will find yourself stepping backwards off your mat in **12**. Either continue or move back to your mat at this point.

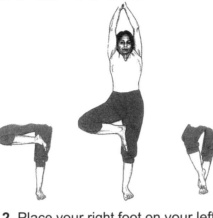

2. Place your right foot on your left thigh. **INHALE** your hands above your head, coming into the **Tree**. Hold for a few breaths.
Observation. Some people have a groove in the thigh where the foot can rest. Others find that the foot slips down. Here are some alternative foot positions.

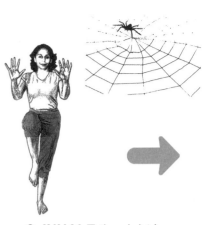

3. INHALE the right knee high in front and lower the hands with the palms facing forwards.

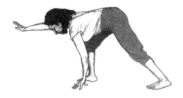

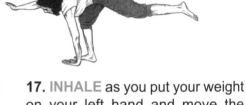

16. When you are ready, **INHALE** round to the front and bend the right knee.
Place your left hand on the floor and stretch your right hand over your head. Hold for a few breaths in a **Diagonal Stretch**, pushing down with your left heel and stretching away with your right hand.

17. INHALE as you put your weight on your left hand and move the shoulders forwards. Lift the left leg and continue to stretch the hand away from the foot.
You can move from **16** to **17** a few times. Push down with your left heel when it touches the floor and feel the stretch on the back of the calf.

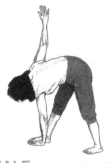

15. EXHALE as you change hands. Lower your left hand to your right foot or the floor and twist round to the right. You can use the same hand variations suggested in **14**.

FOOT ALIGNMENT

SOME yoga teachers prefer this alignment of the feet to the more frequently used alignment. The latter has the back foot turned outwards and the feet are more in line with each other.
Try to keep the hips level.

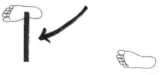

The feet are a hip-width apart

and parallel to each other

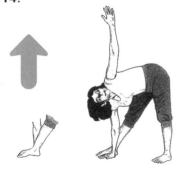

14. Without lifting your head, slide your right hand down your leg. It can rest on the foot or the floor, on either side of the foot. **INHALE** as you lift your left hand and look up.
Keep twisting to the left on the exhalations. You can place your left hand on the left hip. This is a variation of the **Triangle**.

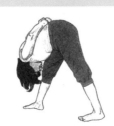

13. INHALE up. **EXHALE** the head down to your right knee.

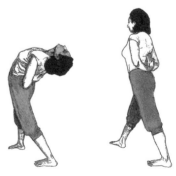

12. INHALE as you step backwards forcefully with your left leg. Try to establish the foot position described above.
EXHALE as you lean backwards.

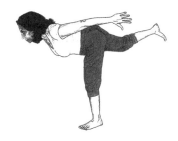

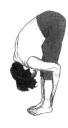

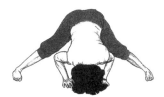

4. EXHALE as you swing your right leg back and the hands into **Flying Bird**.
Look up and hold for a few breaths in the **Swallow**.

5. Soften the knees as you EXHALE into **Standing Forward Bend**.
Hold, breathe and feel the stretch on the lower spine and the backs of your legs.

6. When you are ready, step out wide to the left. EXHALE as you place your hands on the floor, bend your elbows and lower your head. Try to get your head to the floor. If necessary, slide the feet further apart. If you can't reach the floor with your head, lower it as far as you comfortably can.

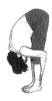

18. Soften the knees as you move your left foot to your right foot, returning to **Standing Forward Bend**.

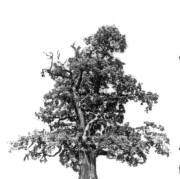

7. Lift your head, press on the hands and move the feet a little closer. With your hands a comfortable distance apart and the feet turned outwards, bend the right knee. Keep lowering to the right until you feel a stretch on the inside of your left leg. Hold and experience the stretch. *Change sides and repeat as many times as you want to*.

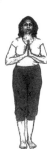

19. INHALE as you return to 1.
Change sides and repeat.

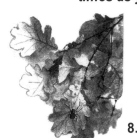

8. Return to the centre. INHALE as you go up on fingertips and tiptoes. The bent knees turn outwards. Bend your elbows and lower your head coming into a **Wide Spider**. Sink into a deep squat and feel the stretch at the top of the thighs.

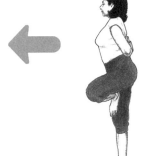

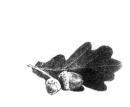

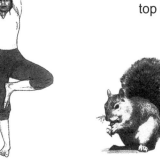

11. EXHALE the hands behind your back in **Prayer**. If that is too demanding, catch hold of your elbows with your hands.

10. INHALE into the **Tree**, with the left foot on the right thigh. Hold for a few breaths.

9. Lower the heels to the floor and move the right foot to the left foot. Return to **1**. This time you will be at the left side of your mat.

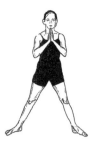

1. Stand with the legs wide and the feet turned outwards. Bring the hands into **Prayer**.

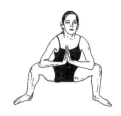

2. INHALE as you sink down into a **Deep Squat**.

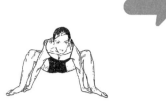

3. Place your hands by your heels with the thumbs on the inside and fingers on the outsides. Sink into a deeper squat.

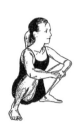

17. INHALE up and stand with the legs wider apart. The toes can be facing forwards or slightly outwards. Sink into a **Wide Indian Squat**. Rest your elbows on your knees and one hand on top of the other. Hold for as long as you want to.

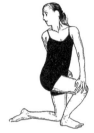

18. Place your left knee on the floor near your right heel. Place your left hand on your right knee and your right hand behind your back. EXHALE as you twist round to the right. *Change sides and repeat.*

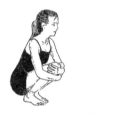

16. Lower your heels to the floor and wrap your hands around your knees. Sink into the **Indian Squat**.

The Squat Sequence

Introduction

THE BREATHING is more obscure in this sequence. You may prefer to exhale into the squats. Hold the postures for as long as you want to and breathe as the body dictates.

Caution: If you have knee problems avoid this sequence.

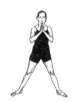

19. Return to **1**.

15. Return to **7**.

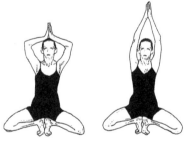

14. Turn the toes outwards with the heels and the balls of the feet touching. Place the hands in **Prayer** on top of the head. INHALE them up and EXHALE them down. *Repeat three times.*

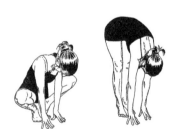

12. Bring the feet together. Go up on tiptoes. Place your fingertips on the floor in front. INHALE as you go into a deep squat. EXHALE as you straighten the legs and arms. *I call this the **Kundalini Frog** as this is the **Frog** as taught in Kundalini Yoga.*
They would suggest doing it dynamically over and over again. Within this sequence do it as many times as you feel you need to.

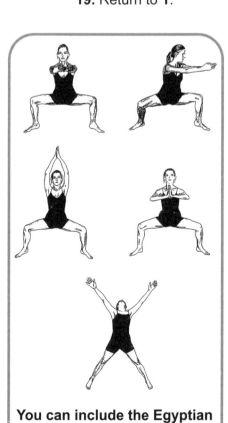

You can include the Egyptian Squats here. They are 16-22 in the Giraffe Sequence.

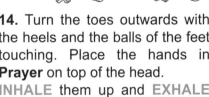

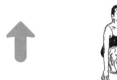

13. Return to **7**.

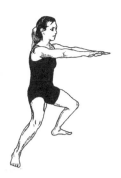

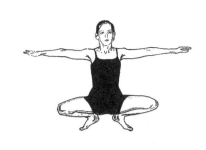

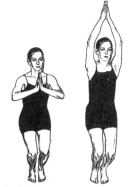

4. INHALE up and extend the arms in front with the palms facing downwards. EXHALE into the **Half Squat**.

5. INHALE up. Bring the feet closer together with the toes pointing outwards. Extend the arms out to the sides. EXHALE into a **Full Squat**.

6. INHALE up. Bring the feet together with the toes pointing forwards. Bring the hands into **Prayer** at the **Heart Centre**. Go up on tiptoes and then bend the knees. Holding the squat, INHALE the hands up and EXHALE them down. **Repeat three times.** This is the **Antelope**.

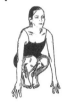

7. EXHALE into a **Full Squat**, still up on tiptoes with the knees forward. Rest the fingertips on the floor.

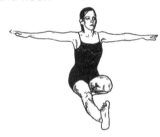

8. Bring your right leg forwards and rest on the heel. INHALE the hands out to the side coming into the **Balancing Squat**.
Change sides and repeat.

Squats in Pairs

AFTER DOING the **Indian Squats** in closed and wide positions, you can try them in pairs.
First, position yourselves an appropriate distance apart. Catch hold of each other with a **Fireman's Lock,** i.e. wrap your hands round each other's wrists. Squat down and, as you lean backwards, pull away from each other.
Try this with the feet together first and then with the feet wider apart.
Hold and enjoy the squats. Come out of the postures carefully. Make sure you don't let go of your partner too quickly and that you help each other come out of the deep squats.

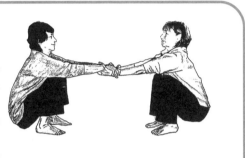

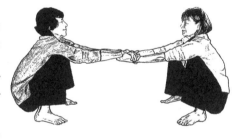

9. Return to **7**.

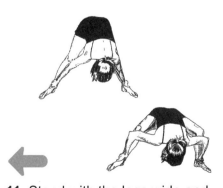

11. Stand with the legs wide and the feet turned outwards. Place your hands on your ankles. INHALE as you bend the elbows and sink into a deep squat. EXHALE as you straighten the legs and arms. **Repeat as many times as you feel you need to.**

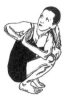

10. Bring the hands into **Prayer** at the **Heart Centre**. EXHALE as you twist your left elbow to your right knee and look up to the right.
Change sides and repeat.

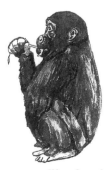

A young gorilla daydreams in the Indian Squat while chewing on a piece of string.

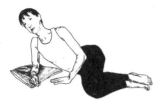
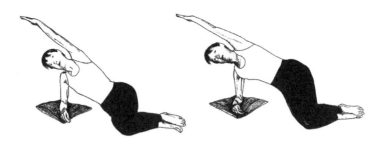

Section 1

1. Place your right forearm on a cushion, as illustrated. The knees are bent to the side. The left hand can rest on the floor.

2. As you INHALE, stretch your left hand over your head. Hold the posture for a few breaths feeling the stretch along the left side of your body.
Now lift the hips and push away with your left hand.

Forearm Rest Sequence

Introduction

IN A class, Swami Ambikananda did postures similar to **3** and **4** in **Section 1**. This gave me the idea of a whole sequence with a forearm on the floor. The ideas kept coming and eventually I divided it up into four sections.

I found it helpful for some pupils with limited mobility. If you have shoulder or neck problems, either avoid the sequence or proceed with caution and stop as soon as there is any discomfort.

The first two and a half sections suggest placing the forearm on a cushion. Doubling up your yoga mat or using a folded blanket is an alternative.

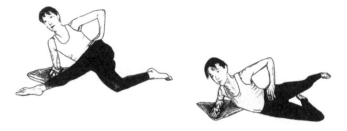

3. Return to **1**. With the hand on the hip, slowly swing your left leg forwards and backwards. Enjoy the sweeping movements. When you swing the leg back, move the chest forwards, stretching the front of your body.
Repeat at least three times.

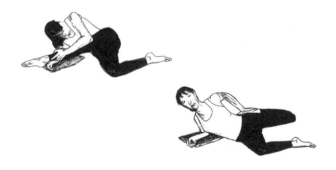

4. Place your left hand on your leg. Swing the leg forwards again. You can bring your head towards your knee.
Now swing your leg back. Change the position of your hand so that you can bend the knee and squeeze the heel into the buttock.

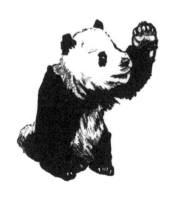

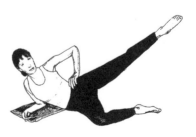

5. Place your hand on your hip and slowly circle the left leg a few times in each direction.
Change sides and repeat from 1 to 5.

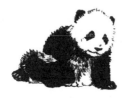

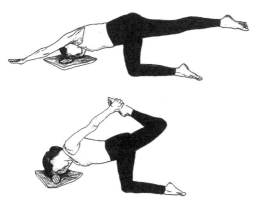

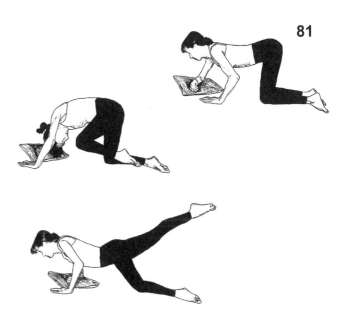

Section 2

1. Come onto all fours and rest your right forearm on the cushion in preparation for a low **Tiger Stretch**. Lift your left arm and right leg. Hold for a few breaths, pushing your left fingers away from your right toes on exhalations.

You can experiment with the position of your head. It can rest on the forearm, be in a neutral position, or you can move your head and shoulders forwards.

When you are ready, catch hold of your right foot with your left hand, coming into a low **Tiger Bow**. Experiment with your head position. Hold for a few breaths.

2. Lower your leg and place your left hand on the floor, as illustrated. Now swing your left leg forwards and bring your head towards your knee. As you INHALE swing the leg back and stretch away with the foot. The leg can be bent or straight. You can move your head and shoulders forwards. Hold for a few breaths. This is a low **Cat Stretch**. *Repeat three times.*

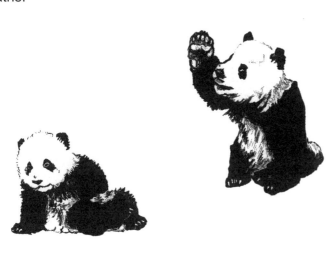

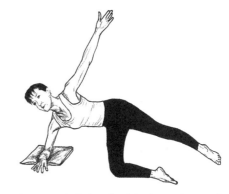

3. Stretch your left leg behind again and then lift your left hand towards the ceiling. If you feel secure, look up at your left hand in a low **Balancing Cat**.

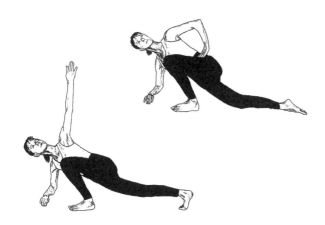

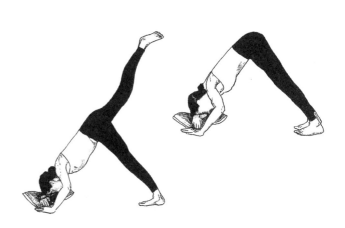

5. Move your left foot forwards bending the knee. Place your left hand on your hip and twist round to the left. Hold for a few breaths.

For a more demanding posture, go up on your right toes and lift your left hand.
Change sides and repeat from 1 to 5.

4. Place your head on your forearm and straighten your legs, coming into a low **Dog** posture. In your own time lift one leg, lower it, and then the other.

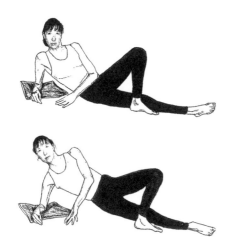

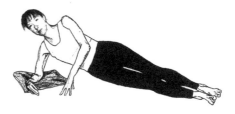

2. Prepare for a low **Side Plank**. Place your left foot on top of your right foot and lift your hips. Either hold for a few breaths or repeat as in **1**.

Section 3

1. With your right forearm on the cushion, straighten your legs out to the side. Bring your left foot over your right leg, as illustrated. Your left hand can rest on the floor.

On the inhalation push on your left foot and lift the hips off the floor. EXHALE them down. *Repeat three times.*

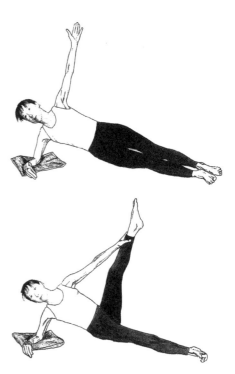

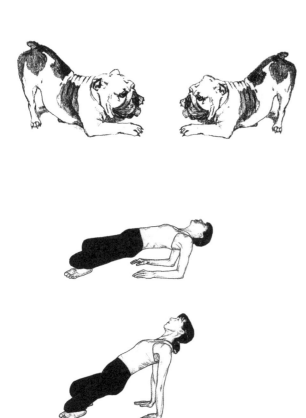

3. Repeat the low **Side Plank** but, this time, lift your left arm.

For a more demanding posture, lift your left leg and catch hold of your foot or leg with your left hand. You can bend the right leg a little and push up on the knee.

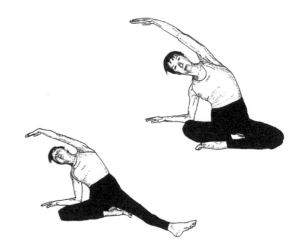

5. Bring your left leg back. Prepare for the **Forearm Backward Bend** by placing both hands on the floor behind. As you INHALE lift the hips. Let your head fall back if it is comfortable. Either EXHALE down and repeat twice more, or hold for a few breaths.

Lower your hips and then place both forearms on the floor behind. As you INHALE lift the hips. Either repeat three times or hold for a few breaths.

Before you repeat the whole of Section 3, repeat 5 with the right foot in front. You will then experience how different it feels with the other foot in front. Afterwards *return to 1, change sides and repeat from 1 to 4.*

4. Sit with your legs crossed in **Easy Pose** and the left leg in front. Lean backwards and place your right forearm behind you on the floor or cushion. Stretch your left arm over your head. Hold for a few breaths, feeling the stretch up the left side of your body.

Now straighten your left leg and push away with your toes. This is an interesting posture to do sitting on a bolster or with the hips slightly raised.

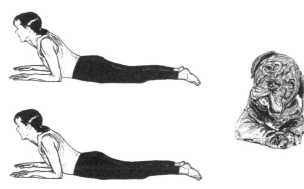

Section 4

1. The **Tilting Sphinx**. Place both forearms on the floor with the fingers pointing forwards. Move the thighs together. The heels can touch if it is comfortable for your back. Move the shoulders down and back.

Some yoga teachers suggest tilting the tail bone downwards and others prefer it tilted upwards. The first method lifts the spine into a **Tabletop** back and the second curves the spine downwards into a **Cat tilt**.

Start by looking downwards, as suggested in the introduction. As you INHALE tilt the tailbone downwards and lift the spine a little. As you EXHALE tilt the tailbone upwards and let the spine move downwards.

Repeat two or three times and then look up and repeat two or three times.

This is a small, subtle movement of the spine.

Introduction

FOR THE whole of this section the height of the shoulders is fixed by the position of the forearms. The movement of the head up and down creates different feelings in the posture.

Experiment by looking down for two or three breaths and then looking up for two or three breaths. You may not like this variation. As with the whole of this sequence, adapt it to suit your needs and preferences.

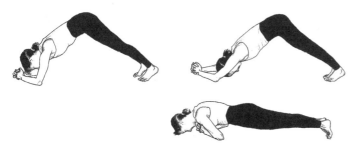

9. With the hands interlocked, move the feet further back until the legs are straight. Swing the head backwards and forwards over the hands in the **Dolphin**. You can try the variation suggested below. If you lift the hands it is easier to get the forehead to the floor in front.

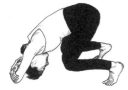 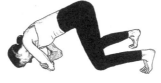

8. Move the feet a little further back. INHALE the head forwards in front of the arms and EXHALE it back. Repeat a few times and then try to get the head to the floor behind the arms and the forehead to the floor in front, as illustrated. This is a variation of **9**.

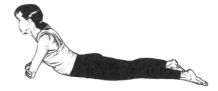

2. Come into a pose similar to the **Cobra** and hold onto your elbows with your hands. The feet can be touching or apart.

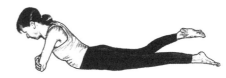

3. Keep the right hip on the floor. INHALE the right leg up and EXHALE it down. Follow the suggestions in the introduction.
Change sides and repeat.

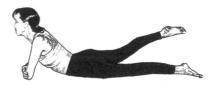

4. Repeat as in **3**, but this time, lift the hip and leg off the floor.

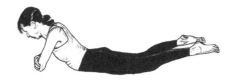

5. INHALE as you lift both legs. Either hold for a few breaths or INHALE up and EXHALE down a few times.

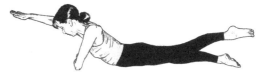

6. Lift your right arm and your left leg. Hold for a few breaths pushing the fingers away from the toes on the exhalations. Experiment with the head positions.
Change sides and repeat.

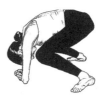

7. Come up on your toes and creep your feet and knees up towards your arms coming into a **Low Spider**. The heels can be up or down.

T3 Sequence

A YOUNG man came to me for private lessons because he had bad back problems. His job involved sitting in front of a computer for many hours a day. Unless he exercised vigorously his back was very painful and problematic.

The postures I have included in this sequence are the ones he found most helpful. When I tried it out with my pupils they liked the way it loosened up their shoulders and upper chest area. Many people have energy blockages and hold tension there and they should find this sequence helpful.

I have called it **T3**, (third thoracic vertebra) because that is roughly the vertebra in-between the shoulder blades. Also it is easy to say and avoids repeating 'the spine between the shoulder blades' throughout the sequence. You can call it **The Computer Nerd Sequence** if you want to.

You need to really concentrate on this particular point, **T3**, when you hold the postures. Do not hurry out of the postures. Hold them and breathe if necessary, until you feel the benefits.

When you push T3 forwards, the sternum will lift up and out. The tail bone will move outwards in the opposite direction.

When you move T3 backwards, the chest will sink downwards and the chin will tuck in. The tail bone will move in the opposite direction, tucking under and moving forwards.

Back   **Front**

Notes on the 12 sections

1. Practise this quite a few times until you have located **T3**, the point you are going to concentrate on, and feel the body moving as described above.

2. The version using the wall can be found in the **Wall** sequence.

3. The first part comes from the **Giraffe** sequence. You need not have your feet so wide apart.

4. This is a mixture of Chi Gung and ideas from different yoga classes.

5. The beginning comes from the **Diver's Posture** sequence. I have added **E** to create the contrasting posture.

6. This is a mixture of the **Crescent Moon** and **Flying Dragon** sequences. I have added **E** to create the contrasting posture.

Continues on Page 85.

T3

7 cervical vertebrae

12 thoracic vertebrae

5 lumbar vertebrae

sacrum of 5 vertebrae
(they are fused together)

coccyx of 4 coccygeal vertebrae
(the tail bone)

**A side view of the spine
showing its natural curves**

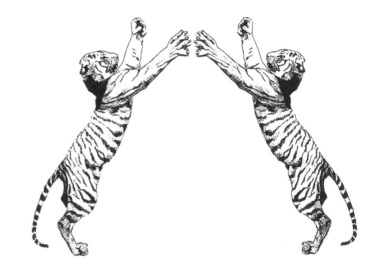

Notes on the 12 sections (continued)

7. This is a simplified version of the **Golden Turtle** from *Iron Shirt Chi Kung* by Mantak Chi, Destiny Books. ISBN: 978-1-59477-04-0

8. I came across the **Camel Ride** in a Kundalini yoga class.

9. My pupil with the bad back found this one very beneficial. For more detail, refer to the **Five Tibetan Rite**s.

10. For more detail and variations refer to the **Diagonal Stretch** sequence.

11. If you find the **High Cobra** too demanding for your lower back, rest on your forearms with the hands pointing forwards. Straighten the left elbow as you twist to the left and vice versa.

12. For more detail about the **Kite**, **A**, go to the **Canoe** sequence.

1

A. Stand with the feet hip-width apart. Place the hands on the hips. As you INHALE lean backwards and squeeze the shoulder blades together. Push **T3** forwards, lifting the chest. Let the head fall back if it is comfortable.

B. As you EXHALE, tuck the tail bone under and slump the back, collapsing the chest and tucking in the chin. Round the shoulders as much as you can.
Repeat slowly about five times.

A   B

2

A. Place your hands on either side of the doorway, with the door open in front of you. This can also be practised on a wall. The feet are further back than the hips. Tilt the tail bone upwards. This lowers the abdomen and lower spine.

Bend the elbows and move the chest forwards. Push **T3** forwards and squeeze the shoulder blades together. Experiment with the height of the hands and tilt of the head until you find the most beneficial posture.

B. Straighten the arms and tuck the tailbone under and tuck in the chin. Push **T3** outwards.

When you have experimented slowly to bring about the most effective movement of **T3**, start to coordinate it with the breath. INHALE forwards and EXHALE backwards.

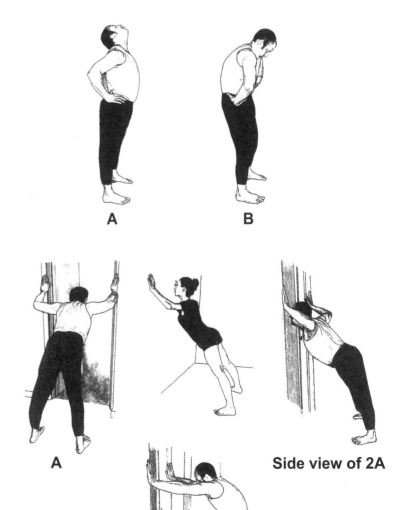

A

Side view of 2A

B

3

A. Stand with the feet fairly wide and the hands in **Prayer**. Roll over onto the outsides of your feet

B. INHALE as you stretch your hands up and out. Look up if it is comfortable.

C. EXHALE your hands to the backs of the thighs. Squeeze the shoulder blades together and push **T3** forwards. Hold and breathe.

D. Move the hands to the sides of the thighs to practise **Star Gazing**. INHALE and then EXHALE as you lower to the right. The right hand slides down the leg and the left hand slides up. INHALE up and EXHALE down to the left. Continue to push **T3** forwards. *Repeat a few times.*

E. For the reverse practice, catch hold of your elbows in front of the body. Push **T3** outwards and tuck the tail bone and chin in. Continue to EXHALE down to the side, and INHALE up, as in **D**. You may choose to soften the knee a little as you lower down to that side. *Repeat a few times.*

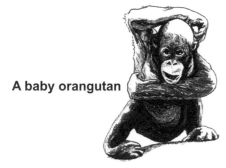

A baby orangutan

4

A. Stand with the feet a little more than hip-width apart. INHALE the hands up with the palms turned inwards. Bring the fingers close together but not touching. Push **T3** outwards and tuck in the chin and tail bone.

B. Go up on your right toes and place your left hand on your left shoulder. EXHALE as you twist round to the right. Look at your right hand. You can adjust the angle of your foot. Bring the shoulder blades together and push **T3** forwards. INHALE back to **A**.
Change sides and repeat as many times as you want to.

C. For a variation, go up on the left toes and twist round to the right and repeat as before. You can also twist round in the opposite direction.

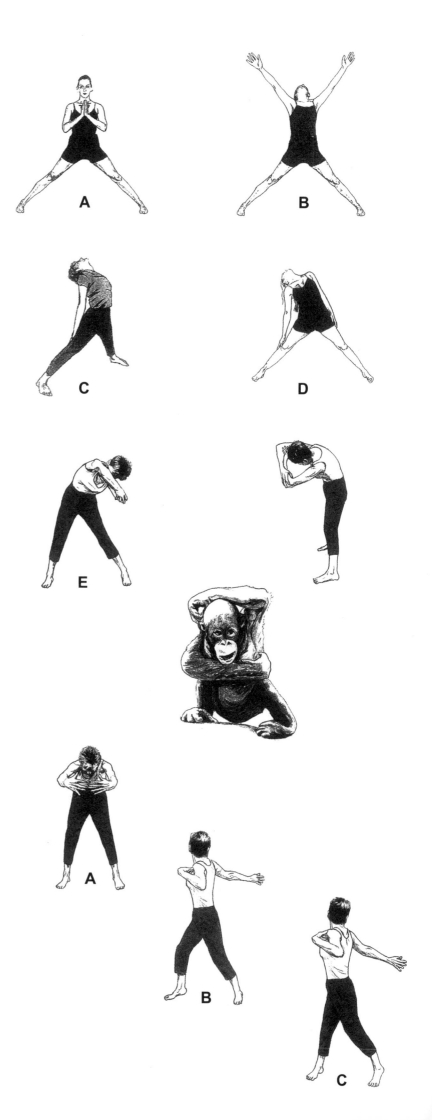

5

A. Stand with the feet together and the hands in **Prayer.**

B. INHALE the hands up above the head and go up on tiptoes.

C. EXHALE into **Diver's Posture**. Swing the hands back in **Flying Bird** and lower the head with the chin forwards. Hold and breathe.

D. Lower the heels to the floor. Bend the knees and INHALE the head up. Sink into a deep squat and lean backwards. Push **T3** forwards, close your eyes and hold for a few breaths.

E. INHALE as you bring the arms forwards and cross the elbows over. Push **T3 outwards**. Hold for a few breaths.

You can repeat the above with the feet wider apart, as described in the **Diver's Posture** sequence.

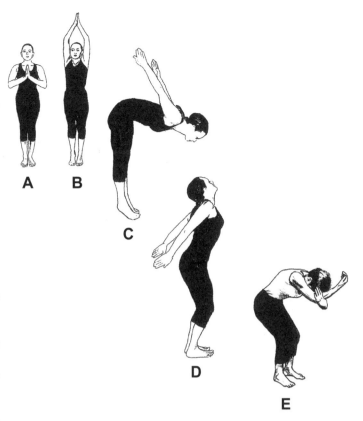

6

A. Kneel with the hands in **Prayer**. INHALE.

B. EXHALE the left foot and hands forwards.

C. INHALE the hands up into **Crescent Moon**. Lean backwards and look up at your hands.

D. EXHALE the arms into **Dragon Wings**. The elbows bend and the palms face upwards. Push **T3** upwards. Hold and breathe.

E. INHALE into the reverse posture. Bring the hands into **Venus Lock** and push the palms forwards. Push **T3** outwards.
Return to A. Change sides and repeat.

F. You can repeat the above moving from a standing pose to **Upward Crescent Moon**. Both knees are bent and you are up on the back toes.

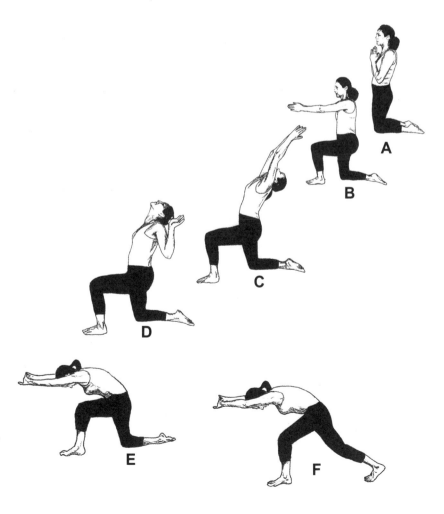

7

A. Stand with the feet hip-width apart and the feet facing forwards. Bend the knees and elbows. Clench the fists with the palms facing upwards, and bring the elbows inside the knees. The back should be parallel to the floor. Lengthen the spine by pushing the tailbone away from the top of the head. This is the **Golden Turtle**.

B. When you are ready, look up and INHALE the elbows up and back. Push **T3** forwards and lift the elbows as high as you can.

C. For the reverse posture, push the clenched fists downwards and lift **T3** upwards.

D. Interlock the fingers under the knees and continue to lift **T3**.
Return to A, passing in reverse order through C and B.

8

A. Sit in **Easy Pose** with the legs lightly crossed. Catch hold of the front ankle with both hands.

B. INHALE as you lean forwards with the elbows low. Push **T3** upwards.

C. EXHALE as you slump backwards. Push **T3** outwards and pull the shoulders forwards. This is the **Camel Ride**.
Repeat a few times and then change the legs over and repeat.

9

A. Practise the **5th Tibetan Rite** (*see page 29*) a few times and then modify the downward posture. Instead of sinking **T3**, which is the usual practice, push it upwards.
  Continue to **Upward Dog** and push **T3** forwards. For the repetitions, INHALE into **Upward Dog** and EXHALE into **Downward Dog**.

B. If you have weak wrists you can practise the above resting on the forearms.

C. You can modify **Dog on a Wall** from the **Wall Sequence** (*see page 118*) in the same way.

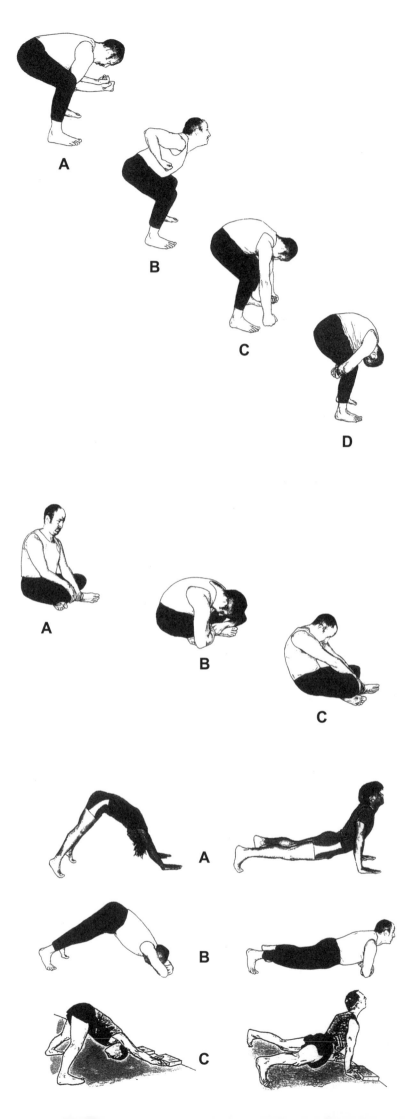

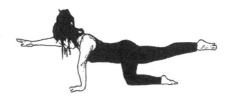

10

You can modify the **Tiger Stretches** (*see page 37*) in the same way.

Start off with the **Tiger Stretch** and progress to the **Tiger Bow**. When you are holding the **Tiger Bow** move the upper shoulder back and push **T3** forwards.
Change sides and repeat.

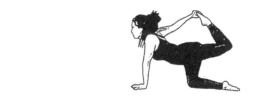

11

A. Lower yourself to the floor and move into a **High Cobra** with the feet comfortably apart.

B. Bend the left elbow and lower the shoulder. Twist round to the right in the **Twisting Cobra**.

This posture helps you to stretch across the shoulder blade area rather than moving it backwards and forwards.
Change sides and repeat.
For the repetitions, INHALE into **High Cobra** and EXHALE into **Twisting Cobra**.

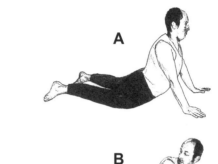

12

A. From the **Stomach Balance** INHALE up into the **Kite.** Hold for a few breaths with the shoulders down and back. The chin can be lifted or in a neutral position, stretching the back of the neck. Hold and breathe.

B. When you are ready, rest on the forearms. Tuck in the chin and push **T3** upwards. Hold and breathe.
Repeat a few times.

C. Roll over onto your back. INHALE as you stretch the hands and feet upwards, lifting the shoulders off the floor. Hold for a few breaths feeling the stretch across the shoulders.
When you are ready, lower the hands and feet and rest in a comfortable position.

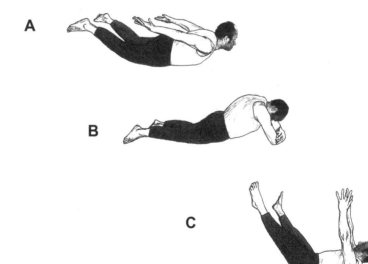

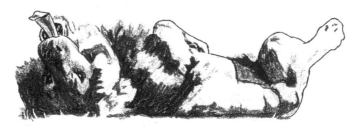

Wide Stretch Sequence

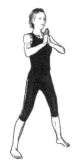

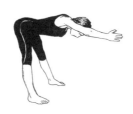

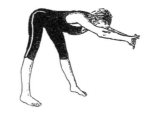

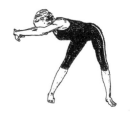

1. Stand with the legs comfortably wide apart and the hands in **Prayer**.

2. **EXHALE** as you lower the head and stretch the hands forwards. Put your weight on the heels and move the hips backwards.

3. **INHALE** as you interlock the fingers in **Venus Lock**. Look down and push away with the palms.

4. **EXHALE** as you twist round to the right.

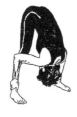

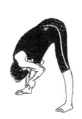

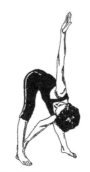

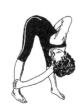

9. Bend your elbows and pull your head and chest towards or through the legs. Hold and breathe, increasing the stretch on the exhalations.

10. Catch hold of your right ankle with both hands.
EXHALE as you bend your elbows and pull your head in to the knee.
Change sides and repeat.

11. With your left hand on the inside of the right ankle, **INHALE** the right hand up. Rotate your right shoulder backwards. Look up at your hand.

12. Move your left hand to the outside of the right leg. Wrap the right hand round your back. Use your left arm to help increase the rotation.
Change sides and repeat 11 and 12.

Mini Leg Raise Sequence

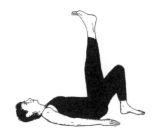

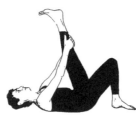

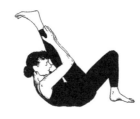

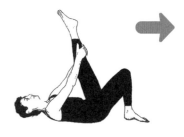

1. Lie on your back with the left knee bent. **INHALE** the right leg up. **EXHALE** it down. *Repeat three times.*

2. Catch hold of the calf with both hands. Ease the leg towards the head on the exhalations.

3. Move your hands further up the leg, bend your elbows and bring the head to the knee. Push the lower spine into the floor. The hips can tilt upwards. Hold for a few breaths.

4. Let your hands slide down the back of your leg as you lower your head to the floor. Point your toes.

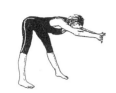

5. INHALE back to the centre.

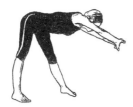

6. EXHALE as you twist round to the left.

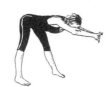

7. INHALE back to the centre. You can add the **Pendulum** here. With the hands on top of the head, EXHALE the head down to a knee. INHALE up and EXHALE down to the other knee. Continue for as long as you want to.

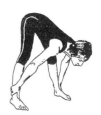

8. Place your hands on the ankles with the thumbs on the front of the legs and the fingers wrapped round the sides.

Go back to page 90

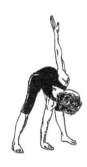

13. Place your right hand on the floor in front. INHALE as you lift your left hand and twist round to the left in the **Twisting Elephant**.

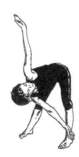

14. Hold the twist and place the back of your right hand on the outside of the left leg. You can place the left hand on the hip and bend the right elbow to increase the rotation.
Change sides and repeat 13 and 14.

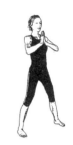

15. Return to **1**.

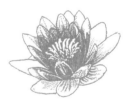

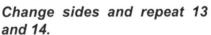

5. Bend your elbows and gradually bring the straight leg towards your head. Increase the stretch on the exhalations.

6. Place the left hand on the left thigh and the right hand, on the inside of the right leg.

Broaden the hips by levering the legs apart. Find the maximum stretch and pause for a few breaths.

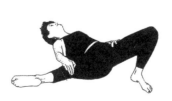

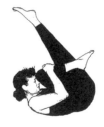

7. Bring your right leg back. Bend the knee, interlock the fingers on top and hug it to you. Stretch the left leg up towards the ceiling with the toes pointed. Bring your head to your knee and rock vigorously.
Change sides and repeat.

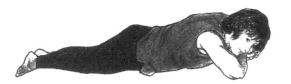

1. Lie face downwards. Place one hand on top of the other and rest the forehead or a cheek on your hands.

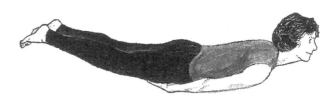

2. Place your hands under the thighs, palms facing upwards. **INHALE** as you lift your head, chest and legs. Gently rock up and down. You will not be able to rock very far.

12. Return to **1** (above), and rest.

The Bow Sequence

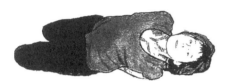

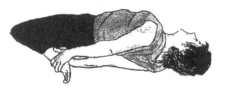

11. Roll from side to side in the **Rolling Bow.**

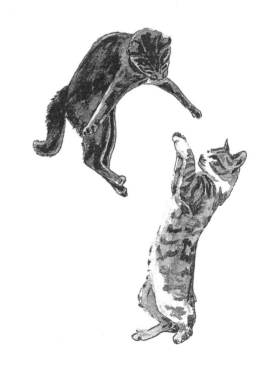

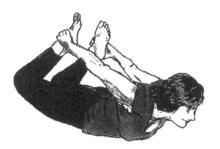

10. Rock up and down in the **Rocking Bow.**

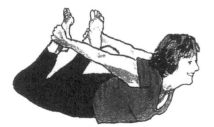

9. Catch hold of both feet with your hands. Separate the knees if necessary. Centre the pelvis into the floor. **INHALE** as you lift the knees, chest and head, coming into the **Bow.**

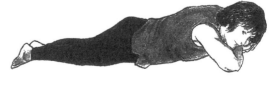

8. Return to **1** if necessary, and rest for a few breaths.

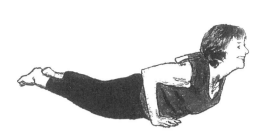

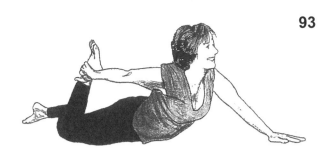

3. Bring your hands close to your waist with the elbows pointing upwards and the fingers forwards. INHALE as you lift the chest, head and legs and rock up and down in the **Rocking Chair**.

4. Catch hold of your right foot with your right hand. Place your left hand on the floor in front. INHALE as you straighten the arm and lift the chest as high as possible. For an easier version, place the left forearm on the floor across the body. Hold and breathe.
Change sides and repeat.

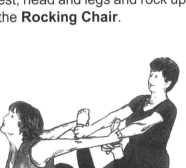

The Bow in Pairs

The helper kneels or stands between the legs of the partner in the **Bow**. They catch hold of the heels on the insides and pull the feet towards them. The partner lets them know when to stop pulling.

This can also be done with the helper standing in the same place and catching hold of the big toes, as illustrated (right), and pulling upwards.

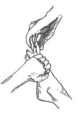

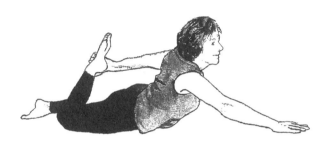

5. Catch hold of your right foot with your left hand. Place your right hand or forearm in front. INHALE as you lift the chest and look up.
Change sides and repeat.

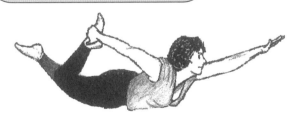

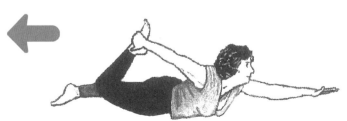

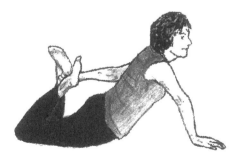

7. Catch hold of your right foot with your right hand. Stretch your left hand forwards. INHALE as you lift the right knee and left hand and look up in the **Extended Bow**. After a few breaths you can lift the left leg.
Change sides and repeat.

6. Cross the feet over. Stretch back with your left hand and catch hold of one of the feet. Experiment with the crossing of the feet. Push up on the right hand or forearm.
Change sides and repeat.

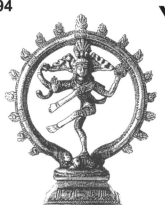
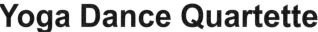
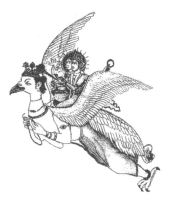
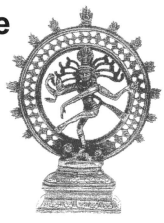

Yoga Dance Quartette

**I am presenting these sequences here in the way they have evolved in my classes.
You may choose to practise them differently.**

I START and finish with the dances of Lord Shiva because they have a simple structure and are easy to learn. In the middle are the Garuda and Krishna dances which have a different flavour. The quartette has become rather like a sandwich with bread on the outside and a contrasting ingredient in the middle.

Sources

I have called sections **1** and **4**, **Nataraja 1** and **2**. Nataraja is another name for Lord Shiva. I came across the first one in a workshop given by Swami Saradananda and the second one in a Dru Yoga workshop. The Dru Yoga School has kindly given me permission to present their interpretation of the posture which is usually called **Lord of the Dance**.

Sections **2** and **3** come from the **Indonesian Flower Dance** as taught by **Warrior Yoga**. Malcolm Bray taught it to me. After the Dutch invasion in 1619 and the subsequent occupation, the villagers were banned from practising their traditional martial arts, Pencan Silat. They disguised their fighting movements in dance and combined them with their spiritual stories which were mainly of Hindu origin.

The Flower Dance is long and difficult to learn. I have selected two sections which seemed both easy to relate to and to teach through illustrations.

Guru Ma Prem (b.1930) left Java after the Japanese occupied the island in 1942. She settled in Holland and formed the Sphinx University where she taught Indonesian arts, martial arts, dance and poetry and eventually Satria Indonesian Yoga (Warrior Yoga).

Notes on Shiva, Krishna and Garuda

The Hindu Trinity is: Brahman the *creator*, Vishnu the *preserver* and Shiva the *destroyer*.

Shiva, often called Lord Shiva, destroys things that are 'past their sell-by date' and makes way for Brahman to start the process of creation again. This process is called the **Cosmic Dance**.

Modern physicists respect and honour this cosmic vision that was intuitively perceived by the ancient yogis during meditation and while in lucid states. In 2004 a two metre high statue of the dancing Shiva was unveiled at CERN, the European Centre for Research in Particle Physics, in Geneva. A special plaque next to the Shiva statue explains the significance of the metaphor of Shiva's cosmic dance with a quotation from Fritjof Capra:

Hundreds of years ago, Indian artists created visual images of dancing Shivas in a beautiful series of bronzes. In our time, physicists have used the most advanced technology to portray the patterns of the cosmic dance. The metaphor of the cosmic dance thus unifies ancient mythology, religious art and modern physics.

Krishna is one of the 10 incarnations of Lord Vishnu or, more simply, God in a human form. The stories of Krishna have their roots in the Vedic age (4500 - 2500 BC). They were transmitted orally and are said to have been written down by Vyasa in about 150 AD. Dates vary greatly.

Garuda is found in Hindu and Buddhist mythology. He is one of the three animal deities. The other two are **Ganesha** (the elephant headed god) and **Hanuman** (the monkey god). Garuda is depicted as having a golden body, white face, red wings and an eagle's beak but a man's body. He has good ethics and corrects evil-doers.

Notes and suggestions

In Warrior Yoga the **Male and Female Hands** position is often used. The hands are in a definite L shape, with the thumbs out to the side and the fingers together. I like to keep my hands in the L shape during these dances as it gives the hands definition. During sections **2** and **3**, I suggest placing the right hand in front when the right leg is raised and the left hand in front when the left leg is raised.

In Section **4** the Dru Yoga School sometimes change the outstretched hand, with the palm facing forwards, to **Chin Mudra**, with the thumb and first finger touching.

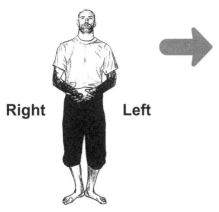

Right   **Left**

1. Stand with the feet together and the feet turned outwards. The hands are on the abdomen with the right hand over the left.

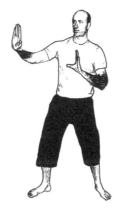

2. Step out to the right with the knee bent and raise your right hand to the side.

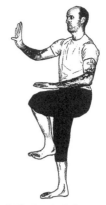

3. Lift the left knee and bring it across the body and let your left hand hover on top with the palm facing downwards.

11. To conclude, return to **1**.

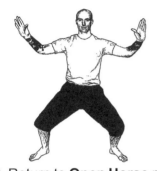

10. Return to **Open Horse** pose, as in **6**.
Repeat as many times as you want to.

Section 1
Nataraja 1

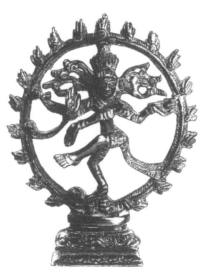

4. Bring the hands together coming into **Lord Shiva's Dance** pose.

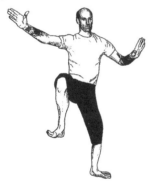

9. Make the semi-circle with your right hand and foot. This is **5** with opposite sides.

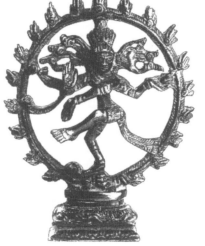

5. Make a large, dynamic semi-circle with your left hand and foot.

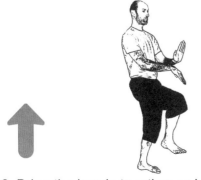

8. Bring the hands together as in **4**.

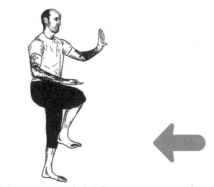

7. Bring your right knee across the body and let the right palm hover over the leg. This is **3** with opposite sides.

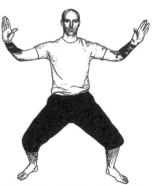

6. Let the left foot land heavily on the floor, coming into **Open Horse** pose.

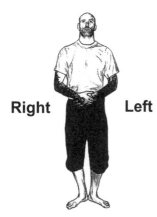

Right   **Left**

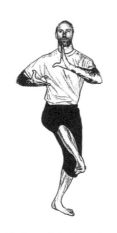

1. Stand with the heels together and the feet turned outwards. Place the hand on the abdomen with the right hand on top. The knees are slightly bent.

2. Lift the right leg keeping the foot flexed. Bring the foot into the centre. Both knees are bent. The hands move into **Heaven and Earth Hands**. The right palm faces upwards and the fingers downwards. The left fingers point upwards.

12. To conclude, return to **1**.

Section 2

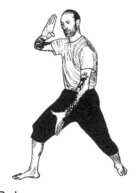

11. Release your arrow as in **6** in **Krishna releases the arrow**.
Repeat as many times as you want to.

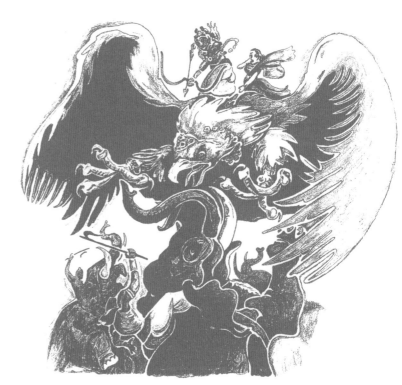

Krishna's Bow

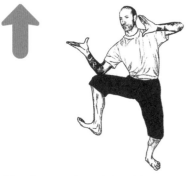

10. Open the right hip as in **5** in **Krishna pulls his arrow back**.

The illustration above was taken from a painting by Rebecca Ann Todd, Madhava Pria.
She kindly gave me permission to copy it. The original is in A4 format with incomplete wings. I have completed the wings.

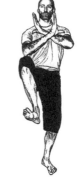

9. Lift the right leg high in front. This is **4** in reverse. The right hand is in front and the right elbow touches the right knee in **Krishna loads his bow**.

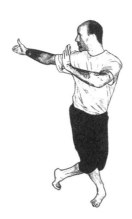

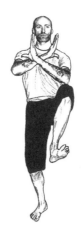

3. Sink the right foot into the floor and raise the left heel. Twist round to the right. Open out the wing completely with the fingers together like feathers. This is **Garuda's Wing**.
Keep twisting round to the right until the right elbow is over the left heel and the left elbow is over the right foot.

4. Rotate back to face forwards and lift the left leg high in front with the foot flexed. Bring the hands into **Male and Female Hands** with the left hand in front. The left elbow touches the left knee. This is Krishna placing the arrow on the bow in **Krishna loads his bow**.

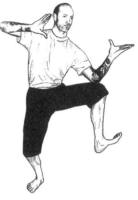

Notes and suggestions

GARUDA plays an important part in the text **Krishna Avatar**. Krishna and one of his wives, Satyabhama, ride on Garuda to kill the evil Narakasura (also called Bhaumasura). On another occasion, Krishna rides on Garuda to save the devotee elephant, Gajendra.

In the **Flower Dance** there is a 180 degree rotation on **6** so that you finish up facing in the opposite direction. The hands also change over. The feet stay in the same place. My simplified version takes up more space. If your space is limited you could try the rotation on **6**.

You can reverse the sequence after **6**, as in **Garuda's Wings**. I have chosen to change sides without reversing.

5. Open the left hip by moving the knee to the left. The leg and elbow maintain contact. At the same time pull your arrow back with your right hand in **Krishna pulls the arrow back**.

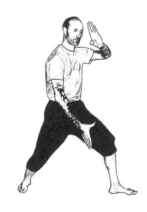

6. To release the arrow lower the left foot to the floor and lift the left hand. At the same time let your right arm swing downwards in a clockwise movement until it comes close to the left leg in **Krishna releases the arrow**.

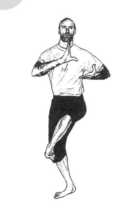

8. Sink the left foot into the floor and twist round to the left. This is **Garuda's Wing** on the other side.

7. Go straight into opposite sides. Put your weight on to the right foot and lift the left leg in front. This is **2** in reverse. The right hand now points to **Heaven** and the left hand to **Earth**.

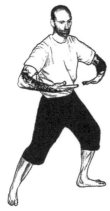

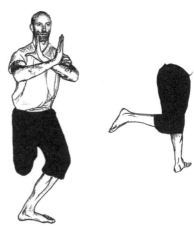

1. Stand with the feet apart, the toes turned outwards and the knees slightly bent. The hands are at waist level with the palms facing upwards in **Garuda folds his wings together**.

2. Bend the right leg. The foot hovers behind at roughly the same height as the knee. At the same time bring the hands into **Male and Female Hands** with the right hand in front.

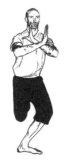

Section 3
Garuda's Wings

Introduction

GARUDA is represented in these statues as the mount or carriage of Lord Vishnu. Garuda is said to have transported Vishnu with him, standing upright on his hands.

When you move from **7** to **5**, you have not dropped your passenger. Garuda has an extra pair of limbs. Your arms and hands change into wings.

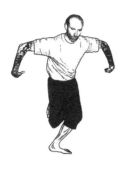

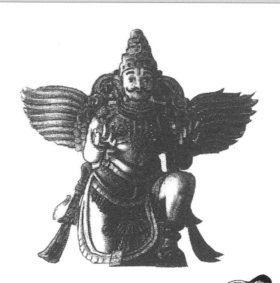

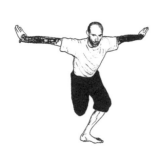

9. Reverse the postures, returning to **1** through **4**, **3** and **2**.
Change sides and repeat.

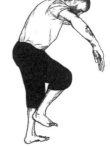

8. When you are ready, prepare to make a large movement. Put your weight onto the front foot and swing up, returning to **5**.

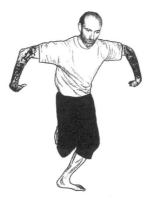

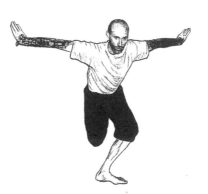

3. Lift the elbows to shoulder height and swing the lower arms back with the palms facing upwards. Look down in **Garuda swings his wings back**.

4. Straighten out your arms to the side with the palms pushing outwards and the fingers (feathers) pointing upwards in **Garuda lifts his wings**. Look up.

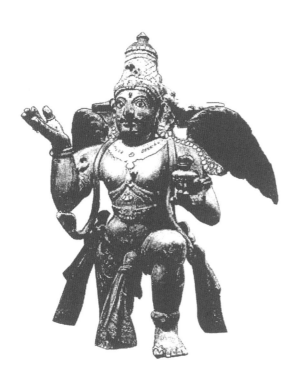

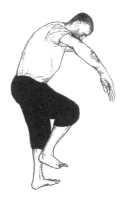

5. Fold your wings forwards and swing your right knee towards your wings in **Garuda folds his wings forwards**.

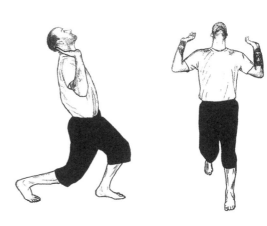

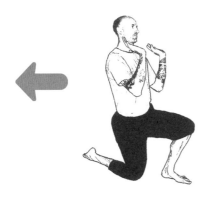

7. Adjust the angle of your back foot and go down slowly onto your right knee, coming into the **Garuda Pose** (as depicted in the statues).
Caution. If you have bad knees, leave out this posture and go from **6** straight back to **5**.

6. Make a large movement with your right leg, stepping backwards onto your toes with both knees bent. At the same time make another large movement backwards with your arms.
With the elbows bent turn the palms to face upwards in **Garuda carries his passenger** (see introduction). Lean backwards if it is comfortable.

Section 4
Nataraja 2

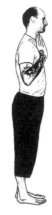

1. Stand with the feet together. Lift your right hand and bring it close to the body with the palm facing forwards.

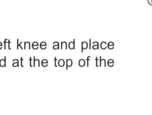

2. Lift the left knee and place the left hand at the top of the thigh.

3. Slide the hand along the thigh to the knee.

4. Continue to slide along the leg. Bring it under the knee and move it along the front of the lower leg until you are catching hold of the foot.

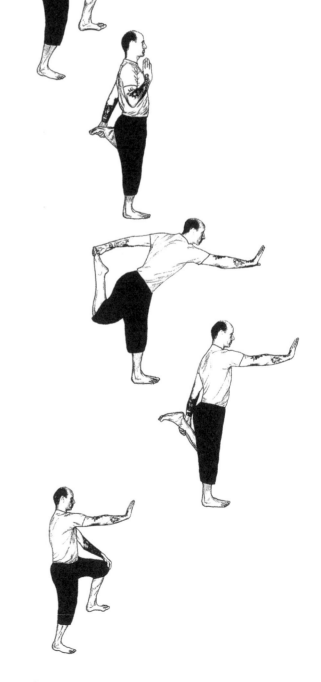

5. Slide the hand up to your toes and lift the left foot behind you. At the same time, push away with your right hand in front and look forwards. Hold for a comfortable duration. This is a variation of **Lord Shiva's Pose**.

6. Slide your hand back along the front of your leg to your knee. This is **2**, **3** and **4** in reverse.

7. When you have returned your hand to the top of the thigh, lower your leg and bring your right hand back. This takes you back to **1**. *Change sides and repeat as many times as you want to.*

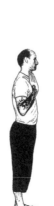

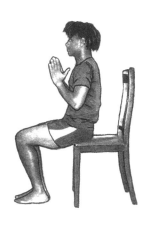

1. Sit at the front of the chair with the hands in **Prayer**.

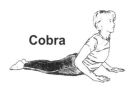

Cobra

The corresponding postures are next to the chair postures. You can practise them first and then their equivalent on the chair.

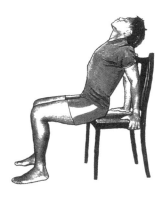

2. Place your hands on the back of the chair seat. **INHALE** as you arch the spine forwards. Let the head fall gently back if it is comfortable. Expand the chest and squeeze the shoulder blades together. Hold and breathe.

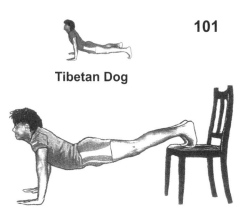

Tibetan Dog

3. Secure the chair against the wall so that it cannot slide backwards. With the body face downwards, place your feet on the chair seat and your hands on the floor, a shoulder-width apart. **INHALE** as you sink the hips downwards and look up.

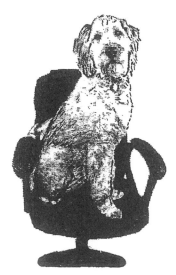

The Chair Sequence

Tibetan Dog

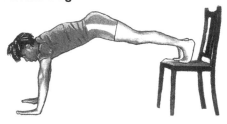

4. EXHALE as you lift the hips as high as you can and lower the head. You can tuck in the chin and bring the head between the arms.
Repeat **3** and **4** as many times as you feel you need to.

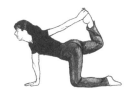

Tiger Bow

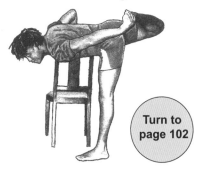

Turn to page 102

7. Catch hold of your right foot with your left hand. Lower your head and lift the foot as high as you can.
Change sides and repeat 6 and 7.

Tiger Stretch

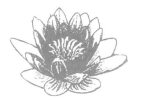

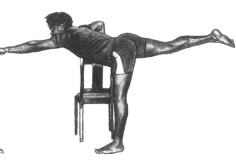

6. Turn the chair around. Stand alongside of the back of the chair with your right hand on top. **INHALE** as you lower the head and lift your left arm and right leg. You may bend the right elbow. Hold and breathe, pushing the fingers away from the toes on the exhalations.

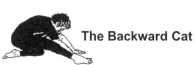

The Backward Cat

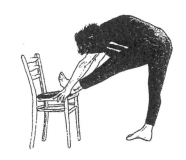

5. Stand a leg distance away from the chair. Place your left heel on the chair and your hands on the seat. Lean backwards with the hips and feel the stretch on the back of your leg.
Change sides and repeat.

102

Lord of the Dance

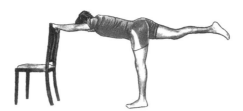

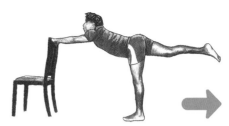

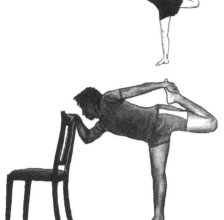

9. Stand a little further back from the chair. Hold the back with both hands. Lower your head and straighten the arms. INHALE the right leg up. Lift the leg as high as you can and lower the chest. Soften the elbows if you need to.

10. INHALE the head up. Hold and breathe, lifting the leg as high as you can.
Change sides and repeat.

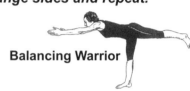

Balancing Warrior

8. Face the back of the chair. Place your right hand on top. Catch hold of your left foot with your left hand. INHALE as you lift the foot as high as you can. You can rest the forehead on your hand if you like.
Hold and lift the knee higher on the exhalations.
Change sides and repeat.

The Chair Sequence (continued)

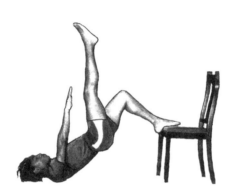

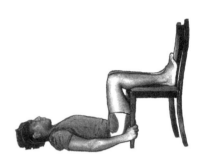

21. Lie on your back with your feet on the chair seat. Catch hold of the chair legs.

20. Experiment by lifting different combinations of legs and hands. You can also make figures of eight with one foot at a time.

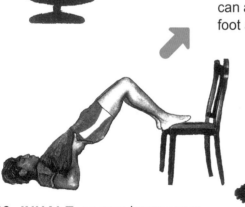

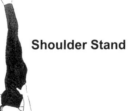

Shoulder Stand

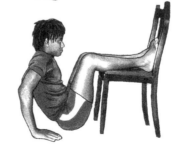

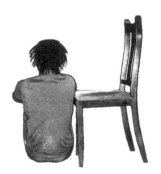

19. INHALE as you lower your head and shoulders to the floor and raise the hips.
Place your hands on the back and the elbows close to your sides.

17. With the chair firmly secured against the wall, sit with your right side against the front of the chair.

18. Swivel round and place your hands behind you, and your feet up on the chair in front.

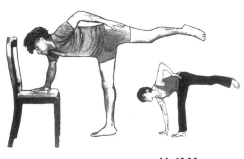

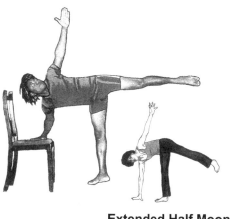

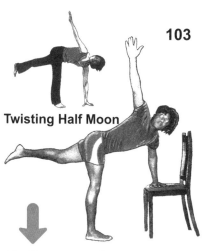

103

Half Moon

Extended Half Moon

Twisting Half Moon

11. Turn the chair around again. Stand in front of the chair and place your right forearm across the seat. You can catch hold of the side of the seat. Lower your head and lift the left leg. Place the left hand on the left hip.

12. INHALE as you lift the left hand up towards the ceiling. Rotate the left shoulder backwards and look up at your hand. Hold and breathe, pushing away in every direction.

13. Keep your legs as they are and change hands. Now with your left hand or forearm on the chair, twist round to the right. Rotate your right shoulder backwards and lift the right hand. Look up at your right hand. Hold and push away.
Change sides and repeat 11,12 and 13.

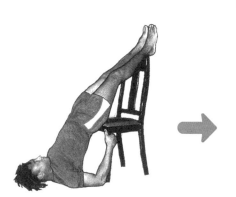

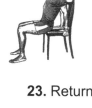

23. Return to **2** and **1**.

Standing Twist

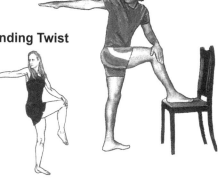

22. Pull the chair towards you and lift the buttocks up on to the chair. Rest your feet on the top of the chair. Keep pulling the chair closer until you are in a comfortable position. You could try meditating in this posture for a short amount of time.

14. Stand in front of the chair. Place your right foot on the seat. With the left hand on the right knee, extend your right arm behind and twist round to the right. Pull the raised knee over to the left and increase the twist on the exhalations.
Change sides and repeat.

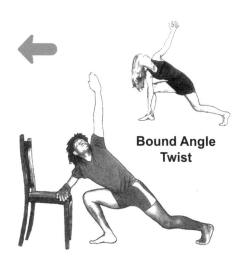

Bound Angle

Bound Angle Twist

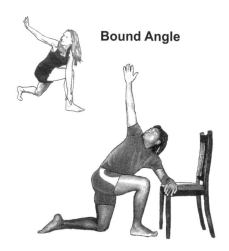

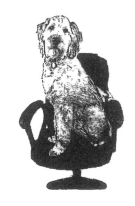

16. Change arms. Lift the left knee off the floor and go up on your toes. Lift your left arm to the ceiling and look up at your hand. If this is too demanding, lower the knee to the floor. Continue to twist round more on the exhalations.
Change sides and repeat 15 and 16.

15. Kneel in front of the chair, with the right foot forwards. Place your left forearm on the seat.
INHALE as you lift your right arm to the ceiling. Rotate the right shoulder backwards and look up at your hand. For a more demanding posture, lift the left knee off the floor as in **16**.

Canoe Sequence

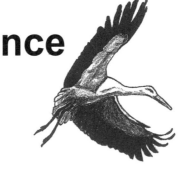

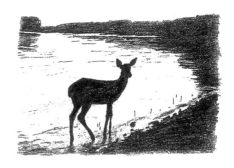

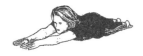

1. Lie on the floor, face downwards with the hands stretched out in front. Every time you EXHALE, push the fingers away from the toes in the **Prone Full Body Stretch.**

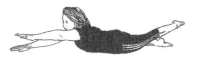

2. INHALE as you raise the left arm and leg. Lift the chest as high as you can and look up. EXHALE them down.
Repeat three times.

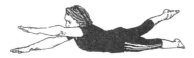

3. INHALE as you lift the left arm and the right leg. For a variation you can put the right hand behind your back. Hold and breathe, pushing way on the exhalations.
Change sides and repeat.

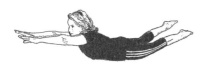

4. INHALE as you lift both arms and legs coming into the **Canoe.** Lift the chest. The chin can either be lifted or tucked in, stretching the back of the neck. Hold and breathe.

5. Roll over onto your right side with the hands above the head in **Prayer.** Rest your right ear on your upper arm. Arch the abdomen forwards and the hands and feet back a little so you are in a banana shape. Stretch away on the exhalations in the **Lateral Full Body Stretch.**

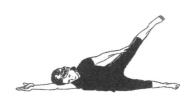

6. Bring your toes towards your head. Press down with the back of your right hand and the side of your right foot. INHALE as you lift the left leg and bring your left hand to the knee in the **Side Snake**. EXHALE them down.
Repeat three times.

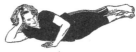

7. Bend your right elbow and rest your head on your hand. Place the left hand on the floor by your side. INHALE as you lift both legs, coming into the **Side Locust**. EXHALE them down.
Repeat three times.

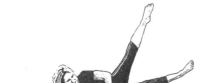

8. Bring your left hand back a little and push up on the finger tips. INHALE as you lift the left leg as high as you can and try to bring the right leg up to it. Push up on the fingertips and hold for a few breaths.

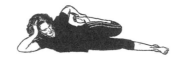

9. Catch hold of your left foot with your left hand. Hold for a few breaths, pulling the leg back on the exhalations and stretching the front of the thigh.

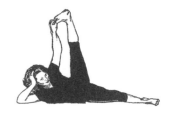

10. Remove the hand from the foot and catch hold of it on the other side of the bent knee. INHALE as you straighten the leg. Hold lower down the leg if necessary. Hold for a few breaths, pulling the leg towards the head on the exhalations.

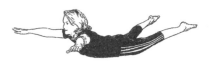

11. Remove the hand from the foot. Roll over onto the abdomen with the hands and feet wide. Hold and breathe in the **Stomach Balance**.

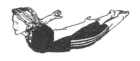

12. EXHALE the big toes together and the hands back in **Flying Bird.** Squeeze the shoulder blades together and lift the chest as high as you can. The chin can be lifted or tucked in as in **4**. This is the **Kite**.

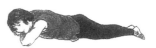

13. Make a pillow of your hands. Rest your head on your hands and bring your awareness to the breath. Observe the movement around the waist. When you are ready, return to **5**.
Change sides and repeat.

The Giraffe Sequence

WHILE LOOKING through 1970's yoga magazines, I was amused to discover that the posture we now call the **Dog** used to be called the **Giraffe**. This was even within the context of **Sun Salutations**.

Possible names for this sequence could have been **Very Wide Leg Stretch** or the **Splits Sequence**. I decided to call it the **Giraffe Sequence** because a giraffe has to stretch its front legs out very wide to drink water or eat grass.

How to breathe in this sequence

I have only indicated obvious breathing patterns needed to get into the postures. Hold them as long as you feel you need to and breathe as the body dictates.

Postures **3**, **13**, **14** and **21** have repetitions. Do not hold these postures. Coordinate them with the breath as indicated.

Caution

It is very important that you 'listen to your body' while doing this sequence. It is demanding and you could hurt yourself if you pushed beyond your capabilities. If you are unfit or have a physical problem, try out a few postures first. Only go through the entire sequence when you are sure it is safe to do so. If you have trouble with a particular posture, leave it out or simplify it.

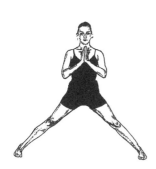

1. Stand with the feet wide apart and the hands in **Prayer** at the **Heart Centre**.

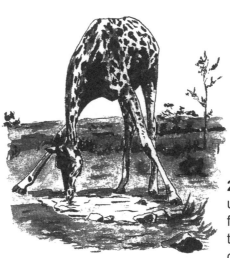

2. INHALE as you stretch the hands up wide over the head. Open out the fingers. Look up at the ceiling with the head back if it is comfortable. Roll over onto the outside of your feet, lifting the inner arch.

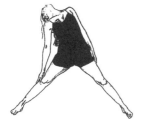

3. Lower the hands to the outside of the thighs into the **Star Gazing** posture. **EXHALE** as you slide your right hand down your leg. **INHALE** up and **EXHALE** down to the left. *Repeat three times.*

4. INHALE back to **1.**

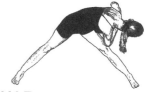

5. EXHALE as you twist round to the left, lowering your right elbow to your left knee
Change sides and repeat.

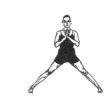

6. INHALE back to **1.**

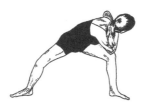

7. Bend your knees and sink down into a deep squat. **EXHALE** as you twist round to the left, lowering your right elbow to your left knee.
Change sides and repeat.

8. Return to **1.**

Turn to page 106

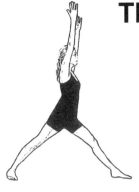

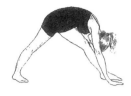

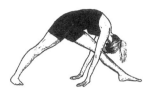

9. Rotate your left foot at a right angle and turn your right foot in a little. **INHALE** as you lift your hands over your head and rotate over your left leg. Separate the hands and stretch upwards. Bring the chest forwards and the arms back.

10. EXHALE as you lower your hands to your ankles or one on either side of your leg on the floor. Lower your head to your knee.

11. Walk your hands backwards with the fingers turned towards the back foot. Lower your head closer to your knees.

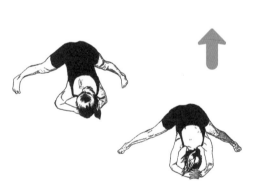

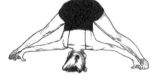

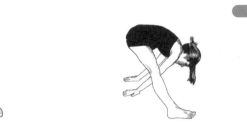

25. INHALE as you come up onto your hands and go up onto your tiptoes and fingertips. **EXHALE** as you bend your knees and sink into the **Wide Spider**. Lower your head and press the shoulder blades together. Sink into a deep squat.

26. Catch hold of your big toes with your first fingers, bend your elbows and lower the head. You may want to widen your stance and put your head to the floor.

27. Walk your hands through your legs with your fingers pointing backwards. Press the fingers into the floor and move the buttocks backwards putting your weight onto your heels. This is the **Backward Elephant**.

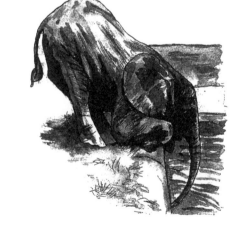

24. Interlock the fingers and swing the head backwards and forwards in the **Wide Dolphin**. If you go right up on tiptoe you may be able to touch the floor with your nose in front of the hands. If you lift the hands it is easier. **Proceed with caution.** Try to touch the floor with your forehead when you swing backwards.

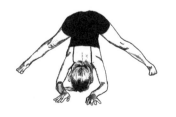

23. Place your hands on the floor and move them forwards into the **Giraffe**. Lower the head to the floor if you can.

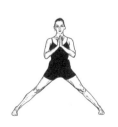

22. Return to **1**.

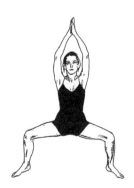

21. INHALE as you raise your hands above your head. **EXHALE** the hands down. *Repeat three times.*

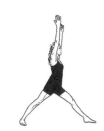

12. Return to **9**.

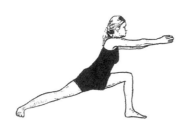

13. Bend your left knee and INHALE as you lunge forwards with your hands in **Prayer**. Go up on the back toes.

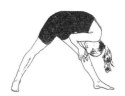

14. EXHALE as you straighten the front knee. Put your hands on either side of the knee. Lower your head to your knee.
Repeat 13 and 14 three times.

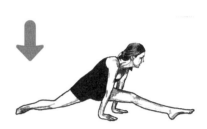

15. Lower your hands to the floor on either side of the front leg. You can rest on the palms or the knuckles. Lower your back knee to the floor. Slide your front foot forwards moving into the **Splits**. Sink down as far as you comfortably can.
Change sides and repeat from 9 to 15.

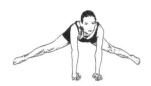

28. Bring your hands in front again and slide the legs out wide into the **Side Splits**. You can slide on the insides of your feet. The soles are off the floor.

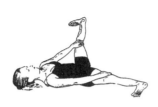

29. Come out of the posture and lie on your back with your legs wide. Place your hands on the backs of your knees, bend your elbows and bring the toes towards the floor in the **Supine Splits**.

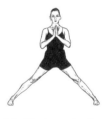

16. Return to **1**.

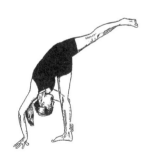

30. Return to **1**. Bring your feet together and lower your hands to the floor. INHALE the right leg up. Place your left hand carefully. You can push up on your fingertips to make a firm base. Wrap your right hand round the calf of your right leg. Bend the elbow and use the arm as a lever to ease your head towards the right knee. Lift the left leg as high as you can in the **Standing Splits**.
Change sides and repeat before returning to 1.

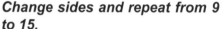

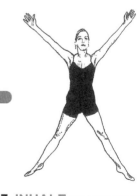

17. INHALE as you go up on tiptoes and stretch your hands out wide. Hold the posture and stretch to the end of every finger.

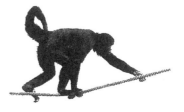

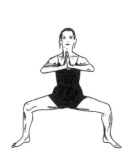

20. Bring your hands into **Prayer** at the **Heart Centre**.

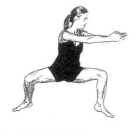

19. EXHALE as you rotate round to the left. INHALE back to the centre and EXHALE as you rotate round to the right.

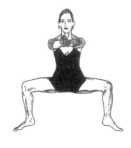

18. INHALE as you bend your knees and bring the hands into **Prayer** in front, coming into the **Egyptian Squat**. Cross the thumbs over. Stay on tiptoes if you can until **22**.

The Haka Dance of the Maori of New Zealand
Adapted for Yoga

Background information

Wikipedia, the free encyclopedia, volunteered this information:

Haka is the traditional dance form of the Maori of New Zealand. It is a posture dance performed by a group, with vigorous movement and stamping of feet with rhythmically shouted accompaniment.

Although the use of haka by the All Blacks rugby team has made one type of haka familiar, it has led to misconceptions. Haka are not exclusively war dances, nor are they only performed by men. Some are performed by women, others by mixed groups, and some simple haka are performed by children. Haka are performed for various reasons; for amusement, as a hearty welcome to distinguished guests, or to acknowledge great achievements or occasions. War haka (peru peru) were originally performed by warriors before battle, proclaiming their strength and prowess in order to intimidate the opposition. Today, haka constitute an integral part of formal or official welcome ceremonies for distinguished visitors and foreign dignitaries, serving to impart a sense of importance to an occasion.

Various actions are employed in the course of a performance, including facial contortions such as showing the whites of the eyes and poking out the tongue, and a wide variety of vigorous body actions such as slapping the hands against the body and stamping the feet. As well as chanted words, a variety of cries and grunts are used. Haka may be understood as a kind of symphony in which parts of the body represent many instruments. The hands, arms, legs, feet, voice, eyes, tongue and the body as a whole combine to express courage, annoyance, joy, or feelings relevant to the purpose of the occasion.

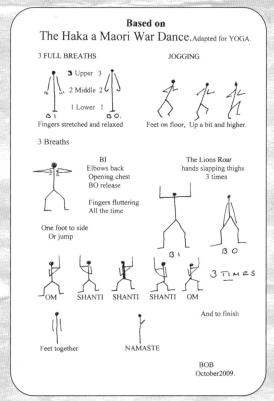

How this sequence evolved

IN OCTOBER 2009 Bob Camp sent me the following A4 document (reduced from A4). I was a bit intimidated by it, but eventually I tried it out with my classes. It needed personal interaction to develop, and comments from pupils have been invaluable.

It is necessary to practise it a few times before you start to appreciate its therapeutic and artistic qualities

One of my pupils, a young osteopath, said it made her feel primitive and tribal. Others have enjoyed using their bodies in different ways and feeling the strange emotions it conjures up.

Although, as stated in *Wikipedia*, the war dance is only one of the art forms of haka, the renderings of the All Blacks New Zealand rugby team have been the major influence in the formation of this sequence. This is because the footage of their videos is so readily accessible. To get the maximum benefit and enjoyment out of this sequence try going to YouTube Haka. There are some very entertaining clips of the All Backs team intimidating the other side before rugby matches.

All the additions to Bob Camp's original version come from the YouTube videos; for example, the puffing out of the cheeks and the placing of the hand on the elbow in **4**. You may come up with your own interpretations and they will be just as valid as mine. I wanted to keep the instructions with the drawings as brief as possible. You will find all the suggestions and alternative interpretations in the notes.

Notes on the postures

1a. Try not to get too involved with the theories of Darwinism and Creationism. This will limit your participation and enjoyment. When you inhale in the **Horse Riding** pose go back a few hundred generations and imagine you were a 'hunter gatherer' and city life not even dreamt of. You can even imagine you were the chimpanzee or gorilla illustrated.

An Indian proverb says *Blessed is the man who can breathe through his bones.* Imagine that you are completely in harmony and in tune with nature and you are breathing in the energy of the cosmos through every pore of your body. You are likely to use a **Ujjayi** breath and the lungs should expand to full capacity. As you do this stretch out the fingers, feel free of limitation and full of potential and power. In this context it can be socially-advantageous or spiritual power rather than physically dominant, aggressive power but you may simply want to feel strong and powerful.

1b. Exhale and curl your fingers inwards. Feel the energy and strength in your hands, and the abdomen flattening as you squeeze the air from the bottom of your lungs. Feel as if you are breathing out through your whole body. You are fearless and part of a powerful group.

2. If you play a stringed instrument you will find this movement of the forearms easy as it is like performing vibrato. The forearm is completely relaxed and you are tilting it, at about a 45-degree angle, from side to side very quickly. The fists are clenched.

Turn the feet outwards. Make groups of four stamps on each side, three times. The first group is a low stamp. The second is a bit higher and the third should be comfortably high. As you stamp your right foot, rotate the right forearm and vice versa. Some people will move the top part of their body a lot when they stamp, others will not need to.

3a. The fluttering of the hands is similar to the rotation of the forearms in **2** but the fists are not clenched. The fingers hang loosely together and the movement of the hand follows the rotation of the forearm.

Feel the feet firmly rooted into planet Earth. As you inhale flutter the hands as far out to the side as you can. Feel the chest broadening out and emulate the feelings you experienced in **1a and 1b**.

3b. Feel as if you are breathing out through your whole body as you flutter your hands back to the centre.

4a and **b.** You can puff out your cheeks after an inhalation and exhalation. It is best to observe the breath, rather than control it, while making these movements. You may not breathe the same way each time you perform them. Keep your feet where they are and just pivot them from side to side.

5a and **b.** You may want to practise the **Lion's Roar**, as described at the beginning of **The Lion's Roar Sequence**, before you try this.

6a,b,c and **d.** This is the usual melody used for this chant. Refer to the **Glossary** for information about the mantra **Om. Shanti** means **peace**.

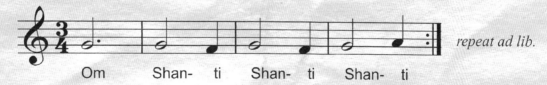

repeat ad lib.

Om   Shan- ti   Shan- ti   Shan- ti

Keep the hands in an **L** shape with the fingers together and the thumbs comfortably away from the fingers. This will add definition to the movements. You may find yourself stamping with the opposite leg to the one in the illustration. Either way is fine. You would only need to do it a particular way if a group of you were performing to an audience.

7. You may say **Namaste** if you like (this means **greetings** and **salutations**) and acknowledge the other members of your group.

The Haka Dance of the Maori of New Zealand
Adapted for Yoga

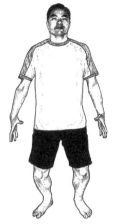

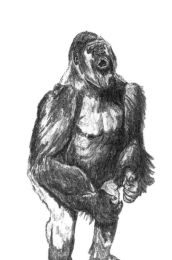

1a. Stand in **Horse Riding** pose. INHALE with a powerful breath into the bottom part of the lungs, and extend your fingers out wide.

1b. Curl your fingers inwards as you EXHALE. Feel the energy in your hands.

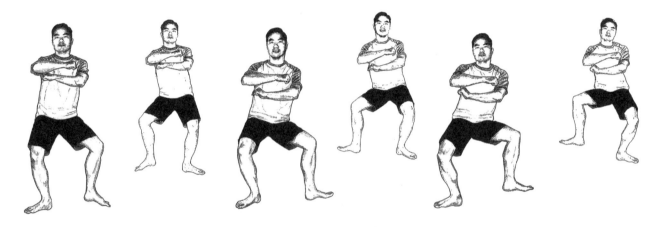

2. Bring the forearms in front of the chest as illustrated, and clench your fists. Rotate the feet outwards. Stamp one foot while rotating the corresponding forearm (as described in the accompanying notes) four times. Repeat on the other side.

Do this three times, starting off with a low stamp and then increasing the height in the repetitions.

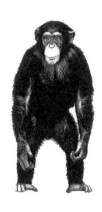

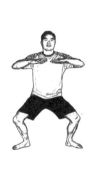

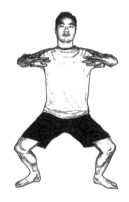

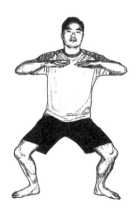

3a. Bring your hands up to chest level with the palms facing downwards. The hands are close but they don't touch. The feet stay still. Start to **flutter** the hands (as described in the accompanying notes). As you INHALE, bring the hands out to the sides, broadening out the chest.

3b. Flutter the hands back to the centre as you EXHALE. *Repeat at least three times.*

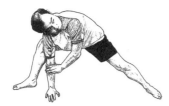 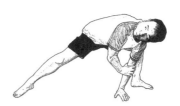

4a. Step out to the right. Bend your right knee and stretch your left foot away to the side. Place your right hand on the floor (more towards the centre than your right foot) and place your left hand on the right elbow. Look up to the left and puff out your cheeks.

4b. Change sides when you are ready. Your breathing is likely to fall into a natural pattern, but if you need help, refer to the accompanying notes.
Repeat at least three times.

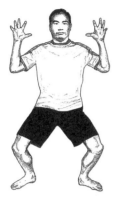 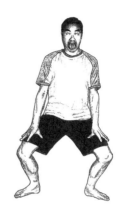

5a. Prepare for the **Lion's Roar. INHALE** deeply through the nose as you bring your hands up. You can curl the fingers inwards to imitate claws.

5b. EXHALE with a **Lion's Roar**. Open your mouth, stick out your tongue and look upwards. At the same time, lower the hands and slap your thighs.
Repeat at least three times.

6. Chant *Om, shanti, shanti, shanti* as you stamp and move your hands from side to side.

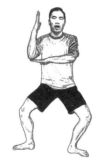 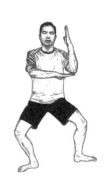

6c. Change again for the second **Shanti.**

6d. Change again for the third **Shanti.**

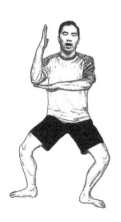

6a. Start with a low stamp. Sing **Om** as you stamp with your right foot and bring the fingers of your left hand to the right elbow.

Repeat this four times.
For the first three repetitions get gradually louder and lift the feet higher (as in 2).
For the fourth repetition, sing softly with a low stamp.

6b. Change sides as you sing the first **Shanti** (this means *peace*).

7. Stand normally with the hands in prayer at the **Heart Centre.**

Repeat the whole sequence as many times as you want to.

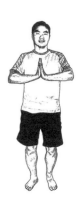

Balance

WE BALANCE by coordinating the messages to the brain from the inner ear, eyes, skin, muscles and tendons.

The inner ear detects the position and rotation of the head. Tiny hairs and fluid within the section illustrated below respond to the force of gravity and monitor activity.

The eyes give visual information about the body's position and further information comes from the skin, muscles and tendons.

If you have difficulty balancing, it is likely to be due to dysfunction in one of the above areas. Do not despair. Just use a few props to give yourself confidence. When you feel confident your concentration will improve. You can press the back or side of one leg against a secure chair or settee. You can hold on to something or use a wall for support.

You are likely to find your sense of balance varies from day to day and that you can balance on one leg better than the other. Staring at a fixed point helps you balance.

Observe what happens to your thinking process when you balance. Try the following posture. You are likely to almost stop breathing or thinking.

Cross one foot over the other and your arms over your chest. Lower your head and close your eyes. The elbows can move away from the body.
Cross hands and feet over the other way and repeat.

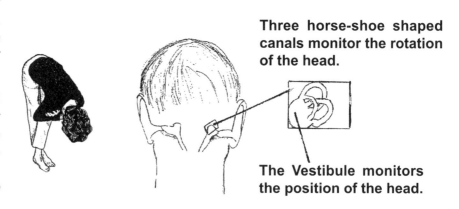

Three horse-shoe shaped canals monitor the rotation of the head.

The Vestibule monitors the position of the head.

The Tree Sequence

THIS SEQUENCE involves standing on one leg for a long time. If you have difficulty balancing, you may want to try it with some support before attempting the whole sequence free-standing.

For maximum support, stand with your hips and shoulders against a wall. Place your right heel about eight inches (20cm) away from the wall as in **A**. This will allow you to lean forward in **4**.

The **Twisting Tree**, **6**, cannot be done with your back against the wall. If you need maximum support, you can do this posture in a doorway so that there is space for your elbows as in **B**.

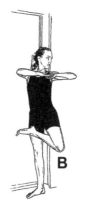

For medium support, a settee or chair seat can be used. Rest the back of the supporting leg on the stable object and place the heel a short distance forward. You can also do the whole sequence with one foot on a chair.

When free-standing, you can either place the left foot at the bottom of the right leg as in **A**, in the **Half Lotus** as in **B**, or high up on the leg as in **1**.

1. Place the left foot on the side of the right leg with the knee out to the side. Your leg may have a natural groove for your foot to rest on or you may have to hunt around for a comfortable position. Avoid wearing trousers with slippery fabric. Bring the hands into **Prayer**.

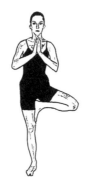

2. INHALE the hands above the head. Straighten the elbows and stretch upwards. **EXHALE** the hands down and **INHALE** them up twice.

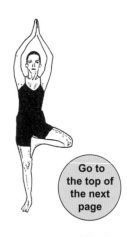

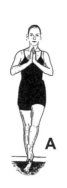

Go to the top of the next page

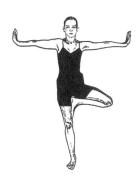

3. INHALE them up a third time. Now **EXHALE** as you 'rainbow' the hands down to the sides with the palms facing outwards. Hold and breathe.

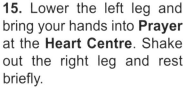
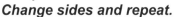

15. Lower the left leg and bring your hands into **Prayer** at the **Heart Centre**. Shake out the right leg and rest briefly.
Change sides and repeat.

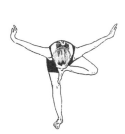

4. EXHALE as you lower your head.

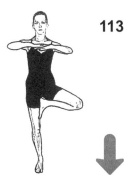

5. INHALE the head up and put your right hand on top of your left hand.

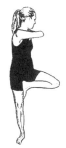

6. EXHALE as you twist round to the left, coming into the **Twisting Tree.**

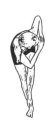

14. EXHALE as you lower the right elbow to the left knee. You may choose to lower the foot down the right leg for this posture or use a wall for support.

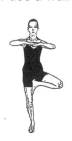

13. INHALE back to the centre.

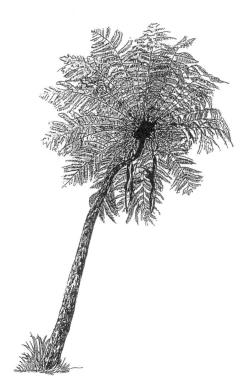

7. INHALE back to the centre.

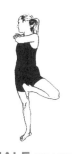

8. EXHALE as you twist round to the right.

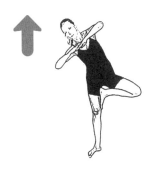

12. EXHALE as you lower the right elbow.

11. INHALE back to the centre.

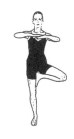

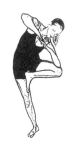

10. EXHALE as you lower the left elbow to the left knee, coming into the **Tree Tilt**.

9. INHALE back to the centre.

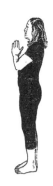

Balancing Prayer

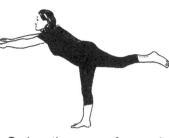

1. Stand with the hands in **Prayer** at the **Heart Centre.**

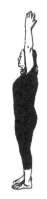

2. INHALE as you stretch the hands upwards.

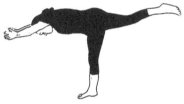

3. EXHALE as you lower the hands and lift your left leg coming into **Balancing Prayer**. Look down at the floor and try to make your arms and leg parallel to the floor.

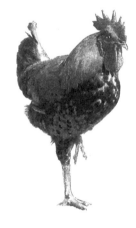

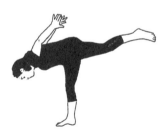

4. INHALE as you swing the hands back in **Flying Bird**.

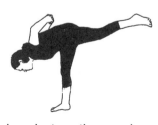

5. Join the hands together and EXHALE as you lower your head and bring the hands up as high as you can. This is **Toppling Tree**.

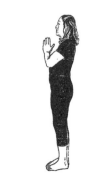

11. Return to **1**.

6. Swing the arms forward and INHALE as you push away with the fingers and lift your head coming into the **Balancing Warrior**.
Change sides and repeat from 1-6.

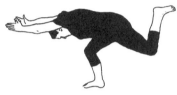

7. Return to **3** but this time bend both knees. You can almost rest the chest on the right thigh. Push the sole of the foot up towards the ceiling.

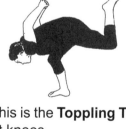

8. This is the same as **4** but with bent knees.

9. This is the **Toppling Tree** with bent knees.

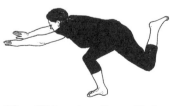

10. This is the **Balancing Warrior** with bent knees. Return to **7**.
Change sides and repeat.

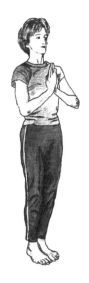

1. Stand with the feet together and the hands in **Prayer**.

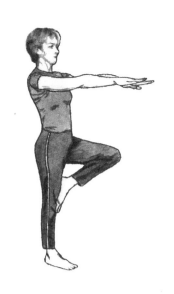

2. Place your left foot on your right knee. INHALE the hands forwards.

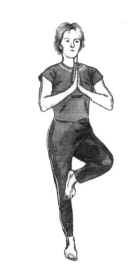

3. EXHALE the hands together.

The Flamingo

Introduction

TO ASSIST your balancing, first try this sequence with the back of the supporting leg against the seat of a chair. Make sure the chair is secured against a wall and can't move.

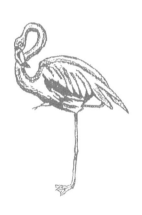

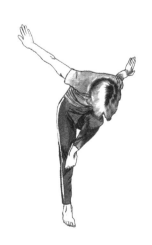

4. INHALE the hands up.
Repeat 3 and 4 three times.

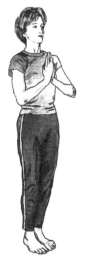

7. Return to **1**.
Change sides and repeat.

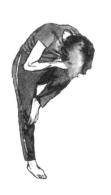

6. Place your right hand on your knee and your left hand on top. EXHALE as you lower your head to your knee.

5. EXHALE your head down to your knee and INHALE the hands into **Flying Bird**.

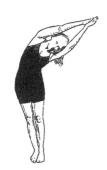
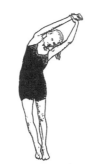
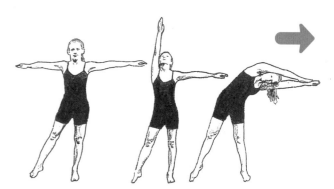

1. This can be done with the feet together or apart. INHALE your hands above your head in **Prayer**. EXHALE them down to the left and swing your hips to the right.
Repeat three times.
Change sides and repeat.
This can also be done on tiptoes and with the hands in **Venus Lock**.

2. Stand with the feet together. Go up on the right toes. INHALE the hands above your head, and catch hold of your right wrist with your left hand. EXHALE as you swing your hips to the right and your hands to the left. Hold for a few breaths, feeling the stretch along your right side. When you are ready, move the hips and hands in the opposite direction and repeat.
Change sides and repeat.

3. Stand with the feet wide and your left foot turned outwards. Lift the hands out to the sides and go up on your right toes. Look at the middle finger of your right hand. INHALE as you bring the right hand up over your head and EXHALE as you lower it on top of your left hand. Hold for a few breaths, pushing the hands over to the left.
Change sides and repeat.

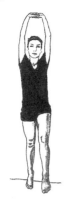

Palm Tree Sequence

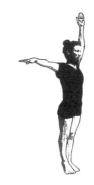
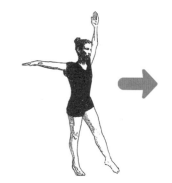

7. Repeat, but this time with your hips and shoulders against a wall. You can bring your leg out to the front and then swing it out to the side.
Change sides and repeat.

8. Come away from the wall and stand with your feet together. Raise your left arm and stretch your right arm out to the side. Lower the shoulders and push away with the fingers. Bring the chin in a little and stretch the top of your head up to the ceiling. INHALE as you lift your left leg as high as you can. EXHALE as you slowly swing the leg to the side and behind. Hold and breathe, lifting the leg as high as you can.
This is the **Holy Fig Tree**.
Repeat, keeping the hands as they are but changing the legs.
Change sides and repeat.

Wall Sequence

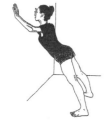
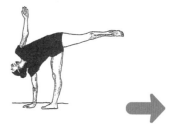

1. Face the wall. Stand a fair distance from the wall, according to your height, with the legs wide and the toes pointing forwards. Place your hands on the wall with the elbows at right angles. Put your spine in **Dog Tilt** (see **Cat Sequence**). Move the chest towards the wall.
Look up and squeeze the shoulder blades together, coming into the **Chicken**. Feel the expansion of the rib cage. You can experiment with lowering the head and putting the spine in **Cat Tilt**.

2. Stand with your back to the wall and your right foot about 9 inches (23 cm) away and parallel to the wall. Bend the right knee a little and lower the right hand to the floor. INHALE as you straighten the right knee and lift the left leg. Swing your shoulders back against the wall and look up. Hold for a few breaths and push away in every direction.
The right palm can press against the wall if you do not want to go down to the floor. **2** and **3** are variations of the **Half Moon** posture.
Change sides and repeat.

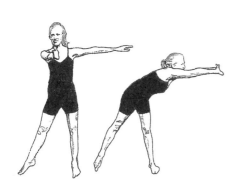
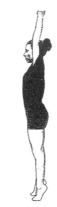
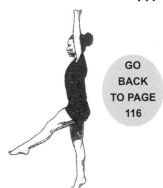

GO BACK TO PAGE 116

4. INHALE as you bring your right hand back the way it came. EXHALE as you slowly swing it in front of the body. Interlock the fingers in **Venus Lock**. Hold and breathe, pushing away to the left as before.
Change sides and repeat.

5. Stand with the feet close together. Interlock the fingers in **Venus Lock** above your head and go up on tiptoes. Hold for a few breaths, stretching upwards.

6. INHALE as you lift your left leg. You can lift it in front or behind. Try to fix your concentration on a point at eye level to help you balance. This is the **Balancing Palm Tree**.
Change sides and repeat.

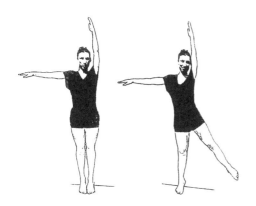

9. Try the **Holy Fig Tree** with your back against the wall, but this time go up on tiptoes.

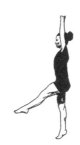

10. Return to **6**, lifting the leg behind or in front, and see if it feels any easier.

The ability to balance varies a lot in this posture. Some days it is easier than others. It helps if you direct all your concentration to the ball of the supporting foot.

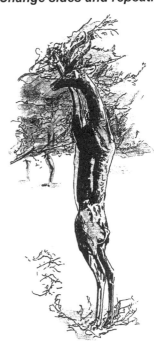

Gazelle Tiptoe Balance

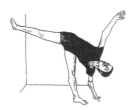

3. Stand a leg's distance away from the wall and place your right foot on the wall at about hip level. The left foot can be at a 45 - 90 degree angle. INHALE as you lower your left hand to the floor, foot or leg and look up at your right hand.

You can experiment by changing hands and twisting round to the left, or catching hold of your leg with both hands and bringing the head to the knee.
Change sides and repeat.

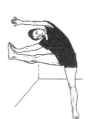

4. Shake out if you need to and return to the same position with your right foot on the wall. Catch hold of your right toes with your right hand. Rotate your left shoulder back and bring your left hand over your head. Try to touch the wall or your foot.
Change sides and repeat.

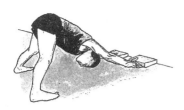
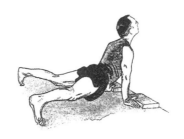
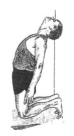

5. In **Dog Against the Wall** you need a block or blocks to create a distance between your hands and the wall so that you can swing forwards. Position your hands comfortably on the blocks and place the feet sufficiently far back and wide for you to sink into a **Low Wide Dog**. Push back on your hands with straight arms and try to get your head to the floor.

6. Swing forwards into an **Upward Dog**, going up on your toes. Repeat **5** and **6** as many times as you want to.

7. With your knees resting on a mat, place the soles of your feet against the wall. Expand the chest forwards and let the head fall back against the wall. Let the arms dangle and the shoulders fall down and back.

Soften the area between the **Heart Centre** and the **Throat Centre**. This area can store depression. Breathe into it love and light.

7 and **8** are variations of the **Camel** posture. You can put something soft between your head and the wall if you like.

Wall Sequence continued

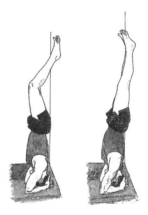

17. If you feel there is too much pressure on your neck, move the hips forwards, bend your knees a little and place the soles of the feet on the wall.

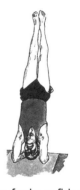

18. If you feel confident and comfortable, move your feet away from the wall.

Hold for a short time at first and slowly build it up to two minutes.

To come out of the posture, return to **16** or lower one leg carefully to the floor and then the other.

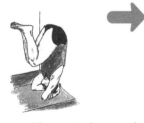

16. To come up with control, use the abdominal muscles to bring the bent knees into the chest. Straighten your legs up to the ceiling and rest your feet against the wall. Not everybody manages to come up like this, no matter how hard they try, and they find their own way. Some bring one leg up first and then kick up with the other one. Others just kick up or ask for help.

13. Headstand against the Wall.
Fold your yoga mat in half and place it against the wall. Your hands are going to cushion your forehead. The little fingers rest on the floor and the thumbs touch the back of your head. The backs of the hands do not rest on the floor. The hands need to be about a hand's length away from the wall. Put your head into your hands and walk the elbows together as closely as possible.

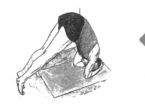

14. Go up on tiptoes. You should feel some pressure on the head but most of your weight should be felt on the elbows. As your back gets closer to the wall, ask an assistant to pull on your elbows. If they come off the floor they are not close enough together or you are not positioned correctly. Do not proceed unless your elbows are digging firmly into the floor.

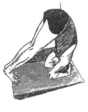

15. Walk your feet towards the wall until your upper back touches, or is close to the wall.

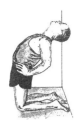

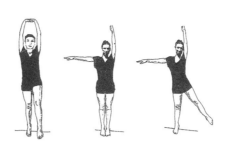

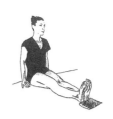

8. Now move a little further away from the wall so that only your toes are touching it. Keep the hips forward, and tilt the head back to the wall. Place your hands on your hips. Continue as in **7**.

You may include part of the Palm Tree Sequence at this point

9. Sit with your back against the wall. Place a book in front of your heels or just take note of the position of your heels.

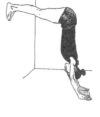

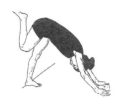

10. Without moving the book, stand up and place your hands along the sides of the book. Line up the base of your hands with the back edge of the book. With your left foot close to the wall, creep the right foot up the wall.

INHALE as you straighten the right leg and bring the left leg up to join it. Push up on your hands. Try to get the trunk and legs as near to a right angle as you can. This is the **Handstand**.

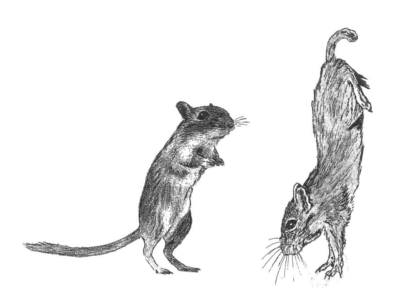

The Gerbil Handstand

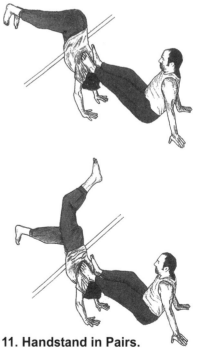

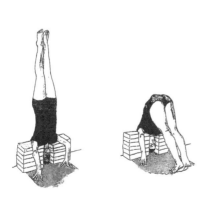

12. Head Stand on Blocks.
Arrange two piles of six yoga blocks on top of each other. Place them against the wall. My illustration shows the long sides of the blocks against the wall but the short side can also be used. They need to be a head width apart (between six and nine inches). You can put a yoga mat under the blocks to prevent slipping.

Place your shoulders on the blocks and your hands on the floor, as illustrated. Keep some distance away from the wall. On tiptoes walk the feet towards your head. When you feel ready, push on the hands and lift the legs up against the wall.

The head should not touch the floor. If it does, put another block on each pile. Stay here for as long as you comfortably can.

11. Handstand in Pairs.
Partner **A** establishes the **Handstand**. Partner **B** sits behind and places their feet on **A**'s shoulder blades. They use sufficient pressure to make **A** feel more secure.

With the help of **B**, **A** will be able to lift one leg up towards the ceiling and then lower it and change legs.

This clever innovation came from a class by Gabi Gillessen.

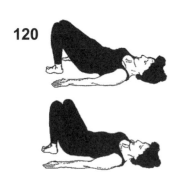
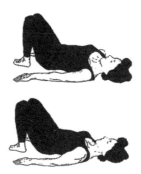
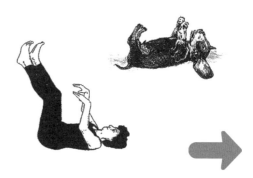

120

1. Dog rubs its back.
Lie on the floor with the knees bent and the feet a hip width apart.
Move your hips from side to side and give your lower back a good scratch.

2. Dog rubs its shoulders.
This time move your shoulders from side to side and give your upper back a good scratch.

3. Very Happy Dog.
Lift your hands and feet up towards the ceiling and give them a good shake.

The Dog Sequence

Introduction
This is another sequence that attracted new postures and expanded. As I have not divided it up into sections, it is necessary to turn to the next page after **121**.

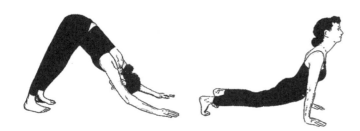

11. Come into **Downward Dog** with the feet further back than usual. Inhale as you swing forwards into **Upward Dog**, as illustrated.
EXHALE back into **Downward Dog**.
Repeat a few times at your own pace.

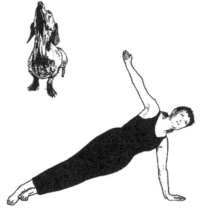

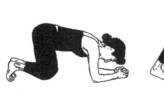

10. Low down Dog.
Return to all fours and lower the elbows to the floor. The palms can be facing downwards or the fingers can be interlocked. As you EXHALE, straighten the legs and go up into a modified **Dog**.
Slowly walk the feet towards the hands and push down with the heels.

9. From **Downward Dog** go into a **High Side Plank**. Move your left foot towards your right foot. Shift your weight on to your left hand. INHALE as you raise your right hand. Hold for a few breaths. EXHALE back into **Downward Dog**.
Change sides and repeat.
Observation. Find a comfortable position for your feet. Some people like to place one foot on top of the other and some like to have both feet on the floor.

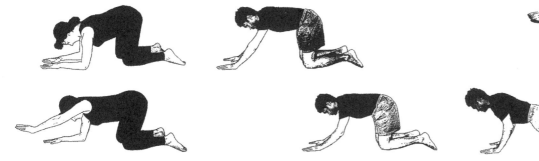

4. Dog shakes its paw.

Come on to all fours and lower the elbows to the floor. Keep the back of the neck long and the shoulders down and back.

Now lift your left arm and stretch the hand forwards. Try to keep the tops of the shoulders level. Hold for a few breaths.

Change sides and repeat.

5. The Dash Hound *(Dachshund)*.

Come back into a **Neutral Cat** (on all fours with a *table top* back) and walk your hands forwards. The hands should be a shoulder width apart. Bend your elbows and tuck them in. Make sure the elbows are in line with the wrists and shoulders.

Move the shoulders forward and hold for a few breaths before going up on the toes and lifting the knees off the floor.

For a more demanding version of the posture, bend the elbows more and lower the nose to the floor

To come out of the posture, reverse the procedure.

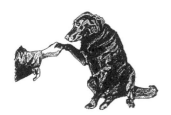
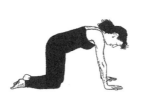
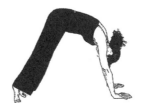
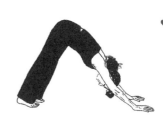

6. Downward Dog.

Come back onto all fours. **INHALE** as you push up on tiptoes and let your head lower between your arms. **EXHALE** as you move the hips backwards and push down with your heels. Walk your feet towards your head until your heels are as low as they comfortably can be.

If you have tight muscles on the backs of your legs you may need to keep your knees slightly bent. Hold the posture for a few breaths. Sink the chest down and back towards your knees, expanding the front of the rib cage.

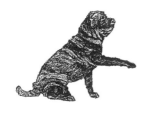
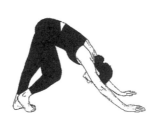
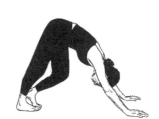

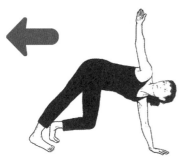

8. Bend your left knee as in **Prancing Dog,** but this time, lift your right arm. Look up at your hand in **Dog lifts its Paw**.

  EXHALE as you return to **Downward Dog**.
Change sides and repeat.

7. Prancing Dog.

From **Downward Dog** push your left heel into the floor and bend your right knee. The heel comes off the floor. Keep pushing down with your left heel. You should feel a stretch on the back of the calf.
Change sides and repeat a few times.

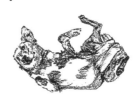

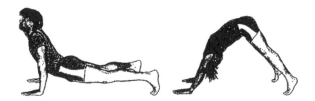 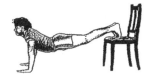 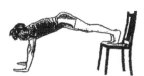

12. The Tibetan Dog.
This is from **The Five Tibetan Rites**. This version is taken from the original drawings found in ***The Eye of Revelation*** (*see page 28*).
No breathing instructions are given.
Go into a **Downward Dog** with the hands a shoulder-width apart and the feet about 2-feet wide and further back than usual.
Go right up on tiptoes. Tuck in the chin and stretch the back of your neck. Hold the posture briefly and tense the Pelvic Floor and as many muscles as you can.
Now swing forwards into **Upward Dog**. Stretch the chin forward. At your lowest point, tense the Pelvic Floor. Repeat a few times.
This is the **Fifth Tibetan Rite.** It would have been repeated 21 times each day.

13. Tibetan Dog on a Chair.
Secure a chair firmly against a wall so it can't slip backwards. Put your feet on the chair and follow the instruction for **12**.
In the downward version you can lift the hips as high as you can and bring your head between your arms.

Partner Dogs

I NEVER really appreciated the **Downward Dog** posture until I practised it in pairs. Try to remember the stretches and sensations you feel when you are being assisted by a partner and then try to reproduce them when holding the posture by yourself.

Partner B assists Partner A.

A can communicate to *B* how far they want to be pushed or pulled and how long they want to hold the posture.

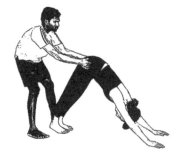
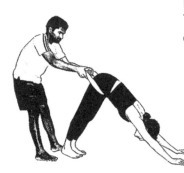

1. *A* is in **Downward Dog**.
B stands behind.
B places their hands on *A*'s hips (the bony parts) and pulls them backwards.
This can also be done with a belt or scarf.

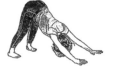 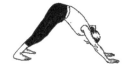 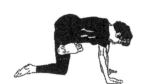

Observation.
There are two basic back shapes in the **Downward Dog**.
Some people have a slight upward arch and some have a downward curve. This has more to do with body type than ability and flexibility.

18. Rovers Revenge.
Come into a **Neutral Cat**. **INHALE** as you lift the right knee to the side, keeping it tightly bent. The left foot is flat. Keep the balance even on both hands and lift the knee as high as you can.
EXHALE the knee down. After you have lifted the knee three times, straighten out the leg to the side. Push the heel away and lift the leg as high as you can. Swing the toes towards your head and hold for a few breaths.
Change sides and repeat.

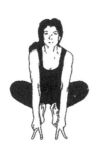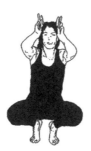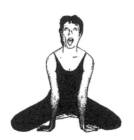

14. Wolf Cub Balance.
Go into a wide squat, on tip toes, with the knees turned outwards. Place your index and middle fingers on the floor.
Hold for a few breaths.
Now place the two fingers on the top of your head to form ears.
Hold for a few breaths.

15. Thirsty Dog.
This is a variation of the **Lion's Roar**. Kneel with the big toes touching and the knees wide.
Place your hands on the floor with the fingers turned towards the thighs.
Now look up and stick out your tongue and make a quick panting noise. This is very good for **diaphragm awareness.**

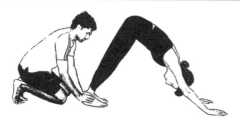

2. B stays behind and kneels down. They place their hands on **A**'s ankles and push them down to the ground.

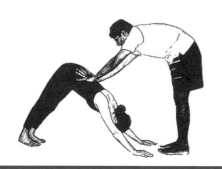

3. B moves round to the front and places their hands on **A**'s lower back and applies appropriate pressure.

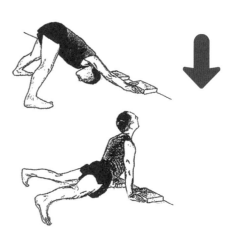

16. Dog against the wall, with blocks.
Place two blocks against the wall a short distance apart. Position your hands comfortably against the blocks and place your feet sufficiently far back and wide for you to sink into a **Long Wide Dog**. Push back on the hands, with straight arms, and try to get your head to the floor.
INHALE as you swing forwards into an **Upward Dog.** Go up on your toes. Repeat a few times.

17. The Dog Stretch.
Sit on the heels in **Extended Child's Pose**. Look forwards and slide your hands away in front until your chest and chin come to rest on the floor. The hips move upwards. The elbows can be straight or slightly bent. Hold for a few breaths.
To come out of the posture, either slide further to lie face downwards or pull the hips back to rest on the heels.

Caution: This is a demanding posture and it will suit some body types more than others. Those who are tall and slim appear to find it most comfortable and beneficial. If you are apprehensive, listen to your body and proceed with caution.

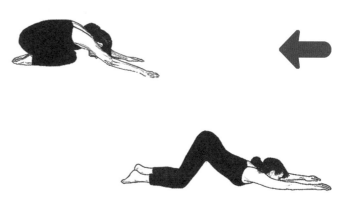

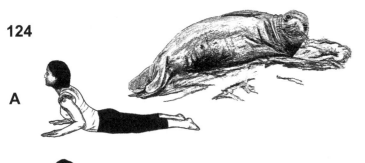

The Seal Roll

A

B

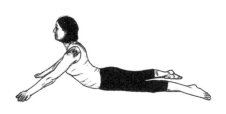

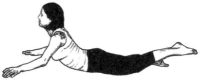

2. Bend your elbows, lowering the chest, and **INHALE** as you lift your left leg. You may rotate your hands forwards.

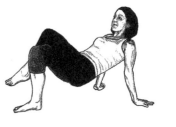

15. Wrap your left leg round the outside of your right leg. Keep the knees close together.

Section 1

1. You can move into the **Seal** pose in two different ways:

a. From the **Cobra** pose, slide your hands forwards, straightening the arms and lifting the chest and abdomen off the floor. Allow your feet to spread apart.

b. Lie face downwards with the feet and hands wide as illustrated. Use your back muscles to lift the chest and abdomen and bring the hands closer to your body. In **Seal** pose your hands are turned outwards.

If you find this posture too demanding for your lower back, use the **Cobra** or **Sphinx** instead and adjust your hand position before moving into **2**.

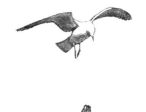

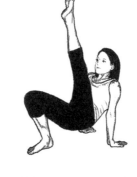

14. EXHALE as you bring your head towards your left knee.

Introduction

THIS SEQUENCE is influenced by the ideas of Sarah Powers and Erling Petersen[1].

It incorporates some postures which are not performed frequently because they do not suit some body types. For example, the **Animal Relaxation** pose and the **Shoelace** pose are more comfortable for those with long arms and legs and narrow thighs. Even the **Sitting Twist** can be awkward for those with wide thighs.

Nevertheless, these postures do become a little more comfortable with practise. Even if you have to invent your own compromise versions, you can benefit through moving your body beyond the boundaries you usually keep.

For example, if you have broad shoulders and short arms you may not get your hands to meet behind your back in the **Cow** but it will still be a beneficial stretch. If you use a strap you can hold the posture and relax.

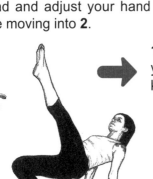

13. Place your hands on the floor behind. With your weight on your hands and right foot, lift the left leg. Stretch it up towards the ceiling with pointed toes.

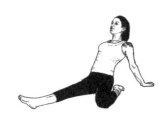

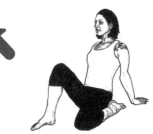

12. Return to **7** and then bring your right foot forwards with the knee bent.

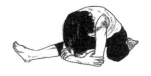

11. INHALE round to the centre and catch hold of your elbows. **EXHALE** as you move them forwards and lower them to the floor. Hold for a few breaths, slowly increasing the stretch.

1. Insight Yoga *by Sarah Powers, Shambhala, 2008. ISBN: 978-1-59030-598-0* Yoga Step by Step *by Erling Petersen, A & C Black, 1984. ISBN: 0-7136-5651-4*

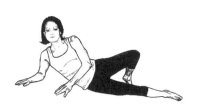

3. Swing your leg over to the right and drop your big toe to the floor.

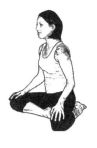

4. Keeping your left foot behind, push on your arms and hands and swing round into **Animal Relaxation** pose. This is a large movement. The right foot stays in front. You will finish up facing in the opposite direction.

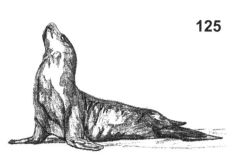

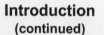

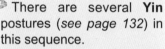

Introduction
(continued)

There are several **Yin** postures (*see page 132*) in this sequence.

Some yoga teachers would consider the **Seal**, **Lying Spinal Twist**, **Seated Twist** and **Shoelace** poses to be **Yin** postures.

You may want to hold them for at least a minute. Depending on your level of fitness and the comfort factor, you can vary the time it takes to move through the **Seal Roll**.

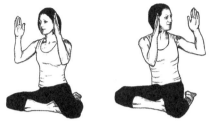

5. After settling yourself in this posture for a few breaths, lift your arms to the side with bent elbows and the palms facing. **EXHALE** as you twist round to the left. **INHALE** back to the centre and then **EXHALE** twisting round to the right. This is an **Egyptian Twist**. *Repeat three times.*

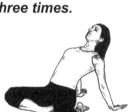

6. Place your hands on the floor behind and lean backwards, squeezing the shoulder blades together.

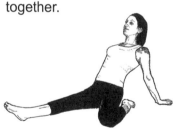

7. Stretch your right leg out to the side retaining the backwards slant.

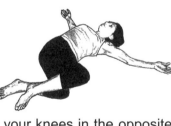

16. Slowly and carefully lower your hips and shoulders to the floor coming into a **Lying Spinal Twist** pose. You can place your right hand on your left knee and apply some pressure. If it is comfortable, you can place the left arm, either bent or straight, beside your head. Hold for a few breaths.
From this posture you can either continue to **Section 2** or proceed back to the **Seal** as suggested below.

17. Swing your knees in the opposite direction.

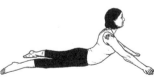

18. With another large movement, roll over to the right and return to the **Seal** pose.
Change sides and repeat.

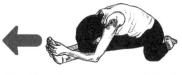

10. Rotate over your right leg and **EXHALE** as you lower your head to your knee. Either hold for a few breaths or repeat three times.

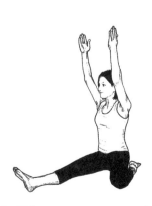

9. When you are ready twist round to the centre and **INHALE** your hands above your head.

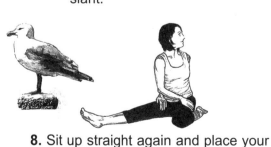

8. Sit up straight again and place your right hand on your left knee and your left hand behind your back. **EXHALE** as you twist round to the left. You may be able to rest your left hand on the right thigh. Hold for a few breaths, twisting round more on the exhalations.

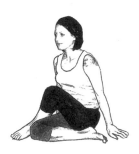

The Seal Roll
(continued)

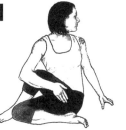

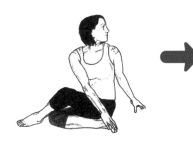

Section 2

1. From **16** in **Section 1**, slowly sit up keeping the left leg on top.

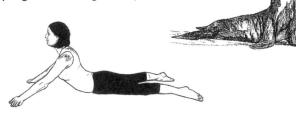

11. When you are ready, lower the legs and roll over onto the abdomen. Return to the **Seal** pose as described in the beginning of **Section 1**.
Change sides and repeat.

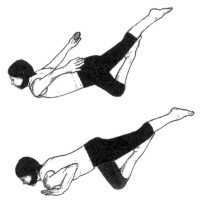

10. Bend the elbows and lower the chest down to the floor. If you are comfortable, you can slide the chest forwards and swing the hands back into **Flying Bird**, coming into the **Dragon Fly**.

9. Place your hands on the floor in front. **INHALE** as you uncross and lift your left leg and go up on your right knee. Place your right foot on the left knee and look up in the **High Dragon Fly**. The spine can be in a **Dog Tilt** or a **Neutral Tilt²**.

Caution: If you have bad knees avoid this posture. Either miss it out and go straight to **10** or return to **16** in **Section 1**, the **Lying Spinal Twist**, and finish in the **Seal** pose as described in **17** and **18** in that section.

2. Prepare for a **Sitting Twist.** Place your left hand on the floor behind and catch hold of your left knee with your right hand or wrap the forearm around it. Lift the chest and on the exhalations pull the left knee to the right and twist round to the left.

For a variation, you can try sliding the left foot forwards and catching hold of the right foot with the right hand.

Hold for a few breaths, twisting round more on the exhalations.

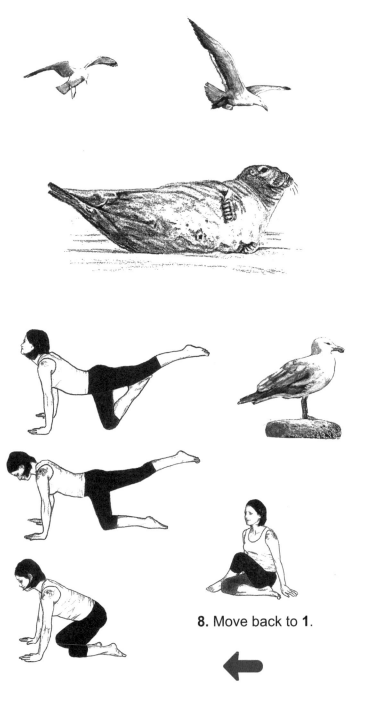

8. Move back to **1**.

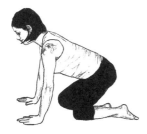

3. INHALE as you twist back to the front and walk your hands forwards. Keep your knees crossed and tightly together.

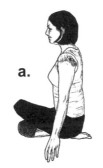 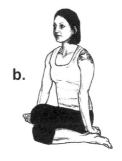 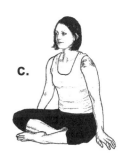

a. b. c.

4. There are three variations here. You may choose the one that is most suitable for your body type, as explained in the introduction.
a. Move the hips back until you are sitting up straight and place the right foot under the anus (in the groove between the buttocks).
b. Come into **Shoelace** pose with both feet out to the side.
First, while the hips are still off the floor, grab hold of both heels and position the buttocks exactly in the middle, between the feet. The weight of the body remains on the hands and feet. Now slowly and carefully lower the hips to the floor.
c. Sit in **Easy Pose** with the legs lightly crossed. You can sit on a cushion or blocks to lift the hips.

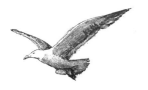 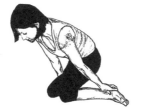

Preparation for the
Shoelace pose

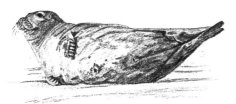

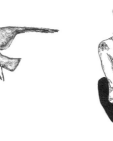

5. When you have established the posture, sit up straight and bring your right hand behind your back. Pull the elbow towards the centre with your left hand.

 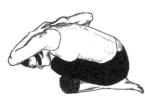 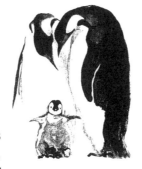

7. When you are ready, **EXHALE** as you lower the head down. If possible, bring your chin in front of your knees or lower the head to the floor. Remember to keep within your comfort zone.

6. INHALE the left hand up, bend the elbow and grasp hold of your right hand. Use a belt or scarf if necessary. Hold for a few breaths, observing your deep breathing. This is **Cow** pose[1].

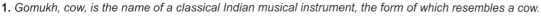

1. *Gomukh, cow, is the name of a classical Indian musical instrument, the form of which resembles a cow.*
2. *In **Dog Tilt** the spine curves downwards. In **Neutral Tilt** the spine flattens like a table top.*

The Swimming Dragon

THIS ANCIENT Chinese Qigong exercise induces a calm, peaceful state of **Pratyahara** (withdrawal of the senses). My pupils love it and some say it is their favourite way of disconnecting from the outside world.

There are several versions of the **Qigong Swimming Dragon**. This one is presented by Philip S. Lansky, M.D. and Dr. Shen Yu (from an article that originally appeared in the American publication *Health World*). They are medical doctors specializing in natural and Chinese medicine. It is considered an 'internal exercise' because it works out and activates **Chi** or **Prana** in the internal organs, muscles, tendons and connective tissue.

It would originally have been practised by monks to enhance health and spirituality. It was gradually incorporated into martial arts and doctors health regimes. This particular version of the **Swimming Dragon** was considered a rapid and powerful method of losing weight.

Qigong divides the metabolism of the body into three **furnaces** or **burners**. The top burner is in the upper chest and controls breathing and the circulation of blood. The middle burner is in the upper abdomen and it regulates digestion. The lower burner is in the lower abdomen. It powers elimination.

The palms are pressed close together and the hands or fingers are used to trace the outline of these three circles. The top and bottom circles are complete but the middle circle is in two halves, one half on the descending path and the other on the ascending path. Another way of thinking about it is one complete circle plus a figure of eight.

The illustrations below show the three furnaces or burners. They also show three neutral positions you will pass through at least twice each time you complete the sequence. For simplicity's sake I have left out the neutral position with the hands above the head.

The feet need to be close together. The palms and the thighs should be pressed tightly together. The hips move in the opposite direction to the hands. It should take about one minute to complete the sequence and it is recommended that you work up to 20 repetitions.

You can practise the sequence in front of a mirror until it is familiar. I prefer to do it with my eyes closed but this may not be how it is usually done. With the senses internalized it becomes a beautiful, peaceful, slow-moving meditation.

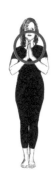

The **Upper Burner** powers the heart and lungs.

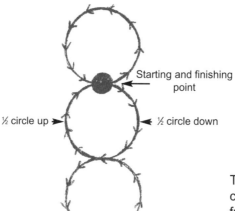

Starting and finishing point

½ circle up ➤   ◄ ½ circle down

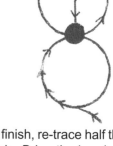

To finish, re-trace half the upper circle. Bring the hands down in front of the face to the **Heart Centre**.
Reconnect to the outside world slowly.

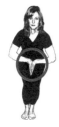

The **Middle Burner** regulates digestion.

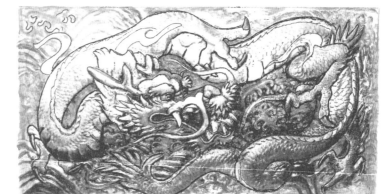

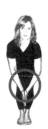

The **Lower Burner** powers elimination.

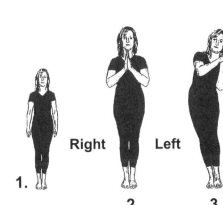
Right **Left**

1.
2.
3.
4.
5.
6.
7.

8.

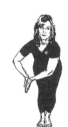
9.

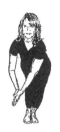
10.

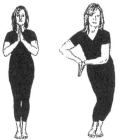
11.

1. Stand with the feet close together and the hands by your side.

2. Press the palms together at the **Heart Centre**.

3. The hands start to circle to the left, passing close to the ear. The head tilts to the left and the hips swing to the right.

4. Circle the hands above the head.

5. As the hands and head move to the right, the hips swing to the left.

6. Pass through **2**.

7. Start to trace the left half of the middle circle. The hands move to the left and the hips to the right. Start to bend the knees.

8. Bend the knees more as you approach the bottom circle.

9. By the time you reach the central position the knees are quite bent.

10. Continue to lower the body as you move the hands to the right and the hips to the left.

11. Continue to circle round to the lowest point.

12. The knees are now bent as much as they comfortably can be.

13. Circle the hands to the left as you swing the hips to the right. Start to straighten the knees very slowly.

14. Continue to circle round to the central point.

15. Pass through **9**.

16. Continue to straighten the knees as you circle the hands to the right and the hips to the left.

17. Continue tracing the circle.

18. Pass through **2**.

To repeat, pass straight through to 3 and 4, then continue.

The Swimming Dragon

18.
17.
16.
15.
14.
13.
12.

Swimming Dragon Variations

THERE ARE many different variations of the **Swimming Dragon**. Some practitioners keep the eyes open and others keep them closed. Some change direction and others don't.

Here are some other examples:

 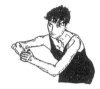

1. The fingers are pointed forwards and the circles are traced with the fingers. The elbows move outwards and the palms are pushed together forcefully. The circles are a little smaller but the hips move more. It has a very Chinese feel about it.

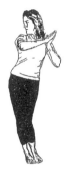 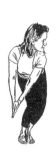 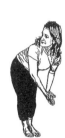

Examples of looking up in the opposite direction to the hands.

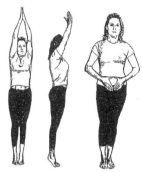

The alternative ending.

2. T.K. Shih expands the **Swimming Dragon** in a delightful way in his book *The Swimming Dragon*[1]. In his version you look up in the opposite direction to the hands. The hips and the head move in the same direction.

To conclude the practice, raise the hands from the **Heart Centre** to above the head and go up on the balls of the feet. After holding briefly, lower the heels and bring the hands to the energy centre in the abdomen. Establish a triangular shape, with the thumbs and first fingers touching. Remain still, till your breathing and heartbeat return to normal. Be aware of exchanges of energy between the palms of the hands and the abdomen. Try to feel subtle movements of energy in the body and perhaps tinglings of energy.

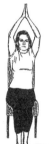 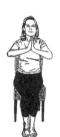 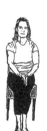 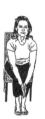 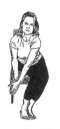 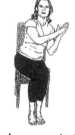

The range of hand movements in the neutral positions.   This shows part of the lower circle.   This shows part of the middle circle.

3. The Seated Swimming Dragon
For those who are confined to a wheelchair, or who are unable to practise the standing version for various reasons, the seated version is an equally magical alternative.

You will need to experiment with the chair you use; e.g., the height, the type of chair seat, soft or hard, and the width. Trace the three circles, as described on the previous page, and add the variations when you are ready.

4. The Swimming Dragon and Meditation
While working on this book, I spent most of one day sitting down in front of my computer or desk.
When it came to my evening meditation, I did not want to sit down again. I decided to try my usual sensory meditation while practising the **Swimming Dragon**. It was such a beneficial experience that I am sharing it with you here.

Breathing Pattern

INHALE at the starting point.
EXHALE as you complete the circle around your head.
INHALE as you do the first half circle of the middle circle.
EXHALE as you complete the bottom circle.
INHALE as you do the other half of the middle circle.

With this pattern you inhale on the middle circle halves and exhale on the upper and lower circles. This makes your exhalations twice as long as your inhalations.

I use my mantra, listen to the inner sound and watch internal colours. I close my eyes and regulate the speed of the practice with my breathing. I continue for at least 10 minutes, or until I feel ready to sit down and meditate.

1, *The Swimming Dragon by T. K. Shih, Station Hill Press. ISBN 0-88268-063-3*
I can confidently predict that devotees of the Swimming Dragon will love this book.

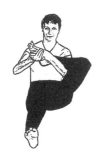

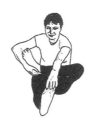

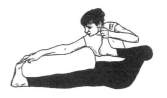

1. Cradle your left foot in both hands. Lift the foot as high as you can.

2. Keep hold of the foot with your right hand. Stretch your left hand forwards to the right foot. Hold and breathe.

3. Catch hold of your left foot with your left hand. Pull it back towards your left ear.
INHALE as you stretch the right hand to the right foot coming into the **Shooting Bow**. Hold and breathe while pulling the foot up and back.

The Shooting Bow

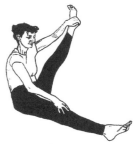

4. Place your right hand on your right knee. With your left hand on your left heel straighten the left leg. You may slump the back a little. Bring the leg back as far as you comfortably can.

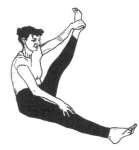

5. Change hands. Catch hold of the left toes with the right hand and lever the left arm under the left knee. Try to get the shoulder under the knee.

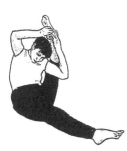

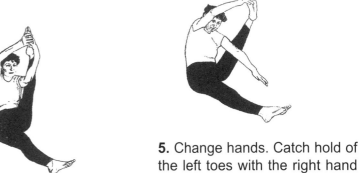

7. Slide the left hand from the side of the foot to the heel or the back of the leg. Try and get the leg over the head. You may want to experiment with hand positions in this posture. You may prefer to put the left arm on top of the leg and catch hold of the toes with the hand.
Change sides and repeat

6. Wrap the left hand round the outside of the left foot and bring the left leg as high and as far back as possible.

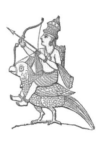

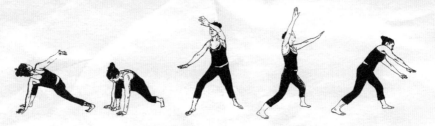

The Yang Sequences of Paul and Suzee Grilley

Paul and Suzee kindly gave me permission to illustrate their three beautiful sequences. They are from their DVD, *Yin Yoga*[1] and they are much appreciated by my pupils. The DVD presents 5½ hours of dynamic, fascinating and, for me, essential information and insight. ***All quotes from the DVD will be in bold italics.***

They made the sequences up themselves. Suzee is a teacher and performer of dance and also a choreographer. Paul studied Taoist Yoga (Chinese Yoga) with martial arts champion Paulie Zink in California, and with Dr. Hiroshi Moyoyama in Japan and the USA.

In the introduction Paul says; ***Yin Yoga is a form of Yoga that stretches and stimulates the connective tissue of the body. It is intended to complement Yang forms of Yoga that stretch and strengthen the muscle tissue of the body. Yin and Yang Yoga are mutually beneficial and both should be practised.***

It is beyond the scope of this book to delve deeply into the theory and practice found in the DVD. I will simply say that in **Yin Yoga** you hold a posture, with the muscles relaxed, for up to about four minutes[2]. In **Yang Yoga** there is a constant flow of movement.

When I first learnt and taught the sequences I split the postures up and paused in-between them to make them easier to learn. When I returned to study them I noticed I had drifted away from the original versions. Suzee demonstrates them on the DVD. She is extremely flexible and flows slowly and gracefully from one pose to another. She takes each pose '*to the max*'; i.e. she stretches or twists into each pose as much as she comfortably can and then slowly glides out of it. She doesn't hold the pose.

Breathing in the three sequences has a similar flow to the movement. It becomes rather like verse 29, Chapter 4 of the *Bhagavad Gita* (Mascara translation, Penguin Pub.). ***Some offer their out-flowing breath into the breath that flows in; and the in-flowing breath into the breath that flows out: they aim at Pranayama, breath-harmony, and the flow of their breath is in peace.***

Something strange happened when I was participating in the *Annual Surya Namaskar-athon* at the Reading Hindu Temple this year[3]. I started doing the **Sun Salutations** as usual, inhaling and exhaling with Ujjayi Breathing in a precise way; e.g. inhale Cobra and exhale Dog. After about my 20th round, I suddenly found myself doing it as if it were a Yang sequence. I didn't split the postures up. I took each pose '*to the max*' and then slowly flowed into the next one. My arms became soft and gentle and it felt quite different. My breathing also changed. The breath just flowed peacefully from one pose to the next. In class my pupils tried doing it the same way and found the changes in sensations very interesting. One of them said, 'That's the way I always felt it should be done.'

It is necessary to know the sequences well before you can move into this continuous flow. In the **Flying Dragon** I have included neutral positions to make it easier to learn. When you are familiar with the sequences you can leave them out, or gently touch the floor with your fingers.

There appears to be some degree of artistic licence when performing these sequences. Suzee does them a little differently each time, e.g. in the **Dragon Swings its Tail** she sometimes stays on the heel and sometimes pushes up on tiptoes (she does the splits in this pose!).

There is a feeling of spontaneity and individual creativity in the sequences and, taking peoples different degrees of mobility and inclinations into account, everybody will do them a little differently. I like my hands to touch the floor in **Dragon Comes Down to Land**. Suzee's hands don't touch the floor. I asked Suzee if that was OK and she said, ***that was a fine variation, as there are several variations of 'coming down to land'.***

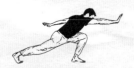

THE YANG SEQUENCES are **The Golden Seed, The Warrior Advances and Retreats** and **The Flying Dragon.** I am presenting the introductions for the Golden Seed and the Flying Dragon here as there is not enough room on their pages. These are Paul's words from the DVD.

Introduction to the Golden Seed

This series of movements is called the Golden Seed. It is a very gentle series of movements that has the advantage that the more the body is warmed up, the more you can work and squeeze the muscles of the, body and so you can work with ease or fairly hard.

The focus is stretching and moving the spine, somewhat stretching the legs, but the focus is the folding, the unfolding and the twisting of the spine. As such, it is a nice series to either start your practice to warm the body up, or to end your practice to cool the body down.

... The important thing to remember in this series, and all the Yang series, is your feet must be mobile. You must feel free to pivot the feet closer together or wider apart as needed. As the sequence of movements becomes familiar to you, some experimentation will tell you exactly how wide apart your feet should be ... You need to adjust your feet very subtly, just before the appropriate movement. With time and experience you will do this naturally, but I want to bring to your attention that your feet are not rooted to the Earth in this series of movements, the Golden Seed.

... Important as any posture is the slow and controlled movement that takes you there. We don't want to do this with momentum, but rather slow the momentum.

Introduction to the Flying Dragon

... It is the most strenuous of the Yang sequences. The reason for that is the body is inverted and the weight is borne on the hands for many movements. The Meridians that stimulate the heart and the lungs are in the arms and so the quickest way to raise the heart beat, temperature of the body and raise the breathing rate, is to strain in a therapeutic way, in a rhythmic way, in a Yang way, the muscles and Meridians of the arms.

So the Flying Dragon works the arms and keeps the body inverted a great deal of the time, which is why it builds the heat and sweat of the body so effectively.

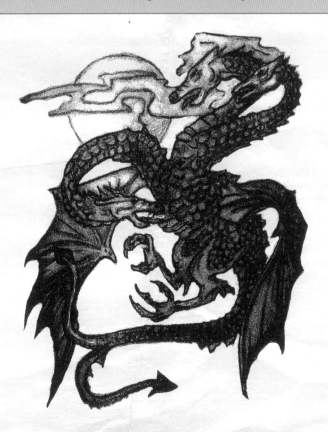

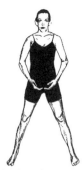

1. Stand with the feet roughly a shoulder width apart and the hands by your sides. Bring your hands to the abdomen with the palms facing upwards.

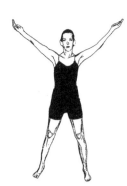

2. *With the inhaling breath, gathering the Chi, bring your hands above your head.*

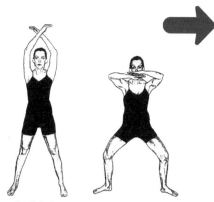

3. Make a loop with your hands by crossing the wrists over and then taking the hands out to the sides. As you do this turn the feet outwards.

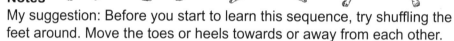

Notes
My suggestion: Before you start to learn this sequence, try shuffling the feet around. Move the toes or heels towards or away from each other.

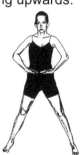

19. Gather the energy at the lower abdomen.
Relax and prepare for the next round. Repeat as many times as you want to.

Variations of hand movements between 10 and 12.

  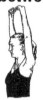

Suzee uses two variations when working by herself.
1. She turns the palms away from the body after reaching the level of the heart. The fingers can be joined or separated. She makes a small circle, in, down and up with her hands and then pushes the palms upwards.

2. She takes her hands behind her head and makes the same kind of circle.
3. When she works in pairs with Paul, they miss out the small circle and take the palms straight up by rotating the palms forward during the ascent.

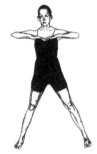

18. Descend the Chi slowly down the body.

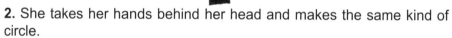

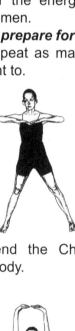

17. Bring the hands above your head with the palms facing downwards.

16. *... release the arms, soften the knees and round the spine as you bring the backs of the hands together.* Connect to the energy of Planet Earth again and draw the Chi up through the backs of your hands as you come up.

15. Swing back into the **Drinking Bird**.

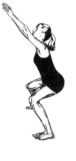

14. *... and then swing the arms forward, lower the hips deep into the Rocking Horse.*

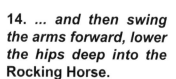

The Golden Seed

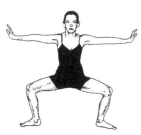

4. Push the palms out to the sides and sink down low into the **Open Horse**. You can lean forwards if you like.

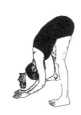

5. Pivot the feet forwards and lower down into the **Elephant Pose**. This stretches the spine and the legs.

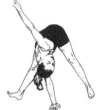

6. Pivot the right foot round to the side on the heel as you lift your left hand, *to get a rotation of the spine and movement of the pelvis as well.*

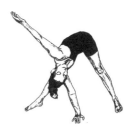

7. As you find your maximum stretch, lower the right foot to the floor.

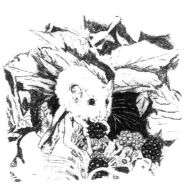

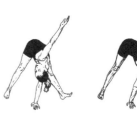

8. Slide your left hand gracefully across the floor to reverse the sides.

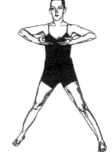

A coconut may be carried for many thousands of miles by ocean currents before germinating on some tropical shore.

The seeds of a blackberry are sufficiently tough to pass through a dormouse without being harmed. This ensures widespread dispersal of seeds.

9. Return, *with smooth control,* to the **Elephant Pose**.

10. Softening the knees and rounding the spine, bring your finger tips to face downwards in front and connect to the energy of Planet Earth. As you slowly stand up, *draw up the Chi from the earth – coiling, rounding and pulling, drawing from the earth with the spine and the legs.*

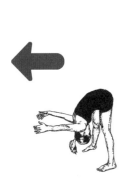

13. Fold forwards, with straight legs and flat back, into the **Drinking Bird**.

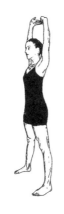

12. Stretch the palms upwards.

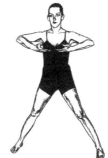

11. *At chest level, reverse the palms and press them upwards, straightening the legs.* Different versions of hand movements between **11** and **12** can be found on the previous page.

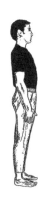
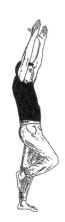
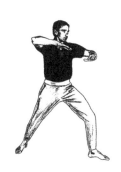

1. Stand with the feet together and the hands loosely by your sides.

2. INHALE as you raise your hands above your head with the palms facing each other, slowly raising your right leg, preparing to move.

3. As you step backwards with your right foot, bring your left hand round in front and start to swing your right hand back.

Warrior Advances and Retreats

AS THE title implies, this sequence is based very much around the **Warrior** pose. It involves *the strengthening and stretching of the legs and the lower body ... so this posture is more about working the legs, the hamstrings, the groin and the thighs.*

The stronger you get and the more warmed up you are, the deeper you can sink into the poses. You can repeat it as many times as you want to ... *building up energy and heat to a greater degree each time you do this routine.*

Modern Meridian Theory

Meridians are the same as Nadis in Yoga. They are energy channels.

This is a simplified version of the **Modem Meridian Theory** as presented by Paul Grilley in his DVD, *Yin Yoga*. His teachers researching the theory are Dr Hiroshi Motoyama, James Oschman and Stephen Birch.

Meridians exist in water-rich phases in the connective tissue. Connective tissue is found all over the body. Life force must travel to every cell of the body. The only tissue that connects every cell of the body is connective tissue.

Veins, arteries, nerves, etc. all have tubes and membranes. Meridians have no membranes and cannot be seen but they can be traced in little spiral granules of HA, **Hyaluronic Acid**.

Meridians have avoided physical detection in the past because scientists did not know what to look for. Research is on-going but, so far, distinct pathways of Hyaluronic Acid have been traced in the skin, which form rivers of energy. These correspond with the established acupuncture points.

Hyaluronic Acid absorbs water. The water wraps itself around the granules. It is a very different system from the Nervous System: *Nerve impulses travel at 180 metres a second. Meridian energy travels at one metre per four seconds.*

All types of yoga posture stimulate Hyaluronic Acid. It is necessary to put appropriate stress on the joints and body components. Without some stress the body degenerates, becomes weak, and the health and energy systems are compromised. Adapting to stress makes us strong.

When astronauts go into space they will lose between 15 and 20 per cent of bone density in a few weeks because they are in a weightless environment and their bones are not being stressed by the pull of gravity.

However, too much stressing of the joints and body components can be very harmful. If yoga is taught and practised with care and sensitivity and with respect for the constitution of each individual, it will stress the body appropriately and well.

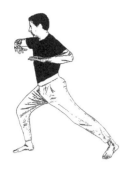

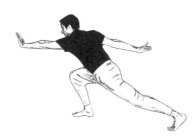

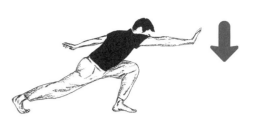

4. Pivot round on your feet so that your right foot is now facing forwards and your left foot is behind you. Your hands continue to circle round.

5. Pushing away with your left hand, lunge over the right leg.

6. *Withdrawing from that, pivoting the feet and lunging over to the left side* ... bring your right hand in front. Stretch the left hand behind and lunge over the left leg. You may extend forwards as far as you choose.

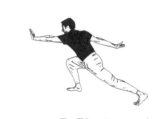

7. Pivot round again and lunge over the right leg, repeating **5.** *You may choose to over-rotate your foot, much like a ballet dancer, for greater stability.*

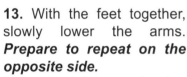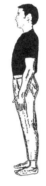

13. With the feet together, slowly lower the arms. *Prepare to repeat on the opposite side.* Raise the left leg and swing the right hand forward. *Change sides and repeat.*

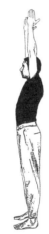

12. *Now swing the arms and torso upwards ... and, using the arms for mechanical advantage,* bring the left foot to the right foot.

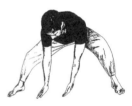

8. *... and then slowly going over to the retreat position, the feet pivot ...* as you glide your hands gracefully along the floor to the left, bending your left knee.

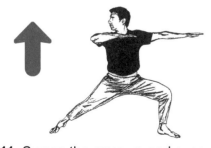

11. Sweep the arms up and over to the opposite side as you pivot the feet again, bending the left knee. *Shift the weight back but this time, keep the weight more upright.* Stretch the arms over to the left and look to the right.

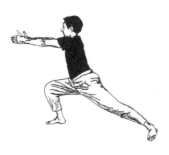

10. *Staying as low as you can, with your strength, move the body forward.* Pivot the feet in the opposite direction so that the right knee is bent. Stretch your arms forward.

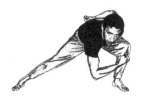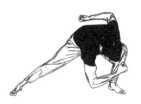

9. Clench your fists. *The right elbow drops down low and the left arm curls back by your ear.*

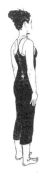 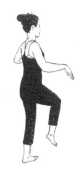 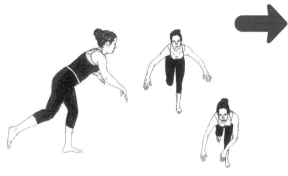

1. Stand at the end of your mat with the feet slightly apart and your hands by your sides.

2. *The dragon starts by slowly unfolding its tail and reaching back.* Lift the arms and the right leg.

3. Extend the right leg back as far as it will go. Lower the leg down on to the toes.

The Flying Dragon

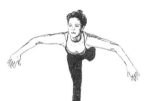 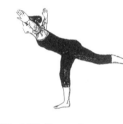 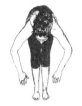 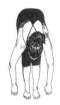

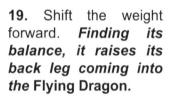

18. Swing the tail forwards coming into a neutral position.

19. Shift the weight forward. *Finding its balance, it raises its back leg coming into the* Flying Dragon.

20. Lift the wings as high as you can and look up.

21. The Dragon Comes Down to Land. Bending the knees, glide the wings down, coming close to the floor.

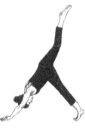

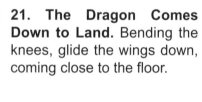

17. Coming back through, pull the leg back to where it was, without touching the floor. Reach up again into **Dragon Swings its Tail**.

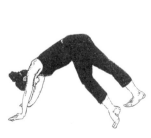 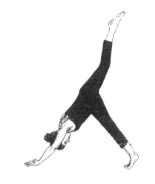

16. *This is* **Belly of the Dragon,** *bearing the weight on one arm, arching and twisting the spine.* Straighten the right leg out, keeping the foot to the floor. Swing the left arm up and back and rotate the belly upwards.

15. *The dragon steps through, swinging the right leg under the body to the left.*

14. Adjust the back leg or hands if necessary as *the Dragon Swings its Tail up behind it, entering into the pose deeply.* Swing the right leg back and up.

13. Slowly return to a neutral position.

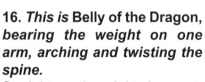

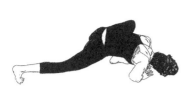 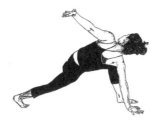 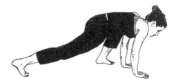

6. Come into a neutral position with both hands forward.

4. *Drop down low onto the arms and legs ... and sink down low into the* Gecko. The back right leg is straight and pressing up from the floor. The head turns to the left.

5. Pressing up, reaching up, and bearing the weight on one arm and twisting with the other to open up the Heart and Lung channels, we reach into **Twisting Dragon.** Straighten the right arm and swing the left arm up and round. Look up to the left.

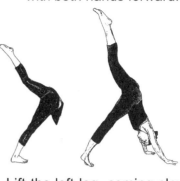

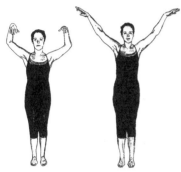 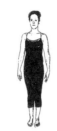

7. Lift the left leg, coming slowly into **Dragon Swings its Tail.** You may need to adjust the back foot or slide the hands back to make the posture comfortable. You can start with the right heel on the floor and then go up on tiptoe.

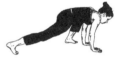

22. *Slowly the dragon unfolds itself. Gracefully sweep the wings up and uncurl them.* Slowly uncurl to a standing position.

23. Lower the wings to your sides, returning to **1**. *Change sides and repeat.* The left leg now extends back into **2**, **3** and **4**.

8. *The dragon raises its tail behind it and then swings its tail forward.* Swing the left leg forwards, coming into another neutral position.

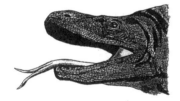

The jaws of a Komodo dragon are powerful enough to bite through metal. The tongue is yellow. In spite of their strength, some dragons in captivity have become so friendly and docile that they are considered safe with young children.

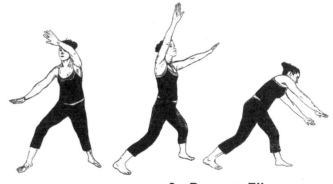

9. **Dragon Flies around the World.** *The dragon flies up and over to the opposite side, pivoting the body and feet.*

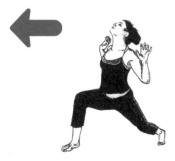 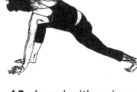

12. *Bring the arms forward and up. At the peak of your attention, bend the arms and contract the scapula, working the arms and the chest and the legs.* Bend backwards and look up, coming into **Dragon Wings**.

11. Return to a neutral position.

10. Land either in another neutral position or on your left hand. Lift the right arm up and back, coming into another **Twisting Dragon**. The right leg is now forward and the left arm is bearing the weight.

Two Birds in a Tree

TWO BIRDS IN A TREE posture can be attributed to Swami Satchidanada Ma. It is inspired by the quotation below, from the *Mundaka Upanishad* (first or second century BC).

I built up a short sequence around it and then added the **Swallow** which came from a workshop given by Ben Parkes. Ben also taught us to do the **Swallow** in a circle, holding hands. We lifted our hands and a knee and then swung the leg and our hands backwards; and then swung the hands and knee forwards again, before lowering them. Ben said his teacher Allan Oakman should take credit for these ideas.

It will enhance your appreciation and enjoyment of this sequence if you are familiar with the quotation and its interpretation found below.

> *There are two birds, two sweet friends, who dwell on the self-same tree.*
> *The one eats the fruit thereof, and the other looks on in silence.*
>
> *The first is the human soul who, resting on the tree, though active, feels sad in his unwisdom.*
> *But on beholding the power and glory of the higher Spirit, he becomes free from sorrow*[1].

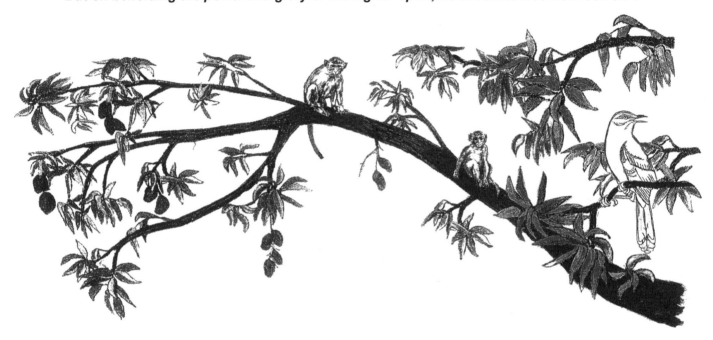

I came across this beautiful interpretation of the above by Swami Gnaneswarananda[2] in a book on meditation by monks of the Ramakrishna Order.

'The sense of fatigue, disgust or depression of the mind comes only because of a psychological confusion under which we are labouring every moment. This confusion is caused by the miscomprehension of the subject and object, the **I** and the **not I**. It is the **not I** which is active, which is doing everything, and which is moving to and fro in this world of phenomena. The real **I** is the witness; it is the illuminator. It takes no active part in any of the functions, either of the body or the mind, save and except illuminating them by means of its innate radiance.

'The moment we are able to distinguish in consciousness between the **I** and the **not I**, the **I**, or 'the subject', at once experiences release, rest and tranquility. This surprising fact needs particular emphasis. Is it not rather strange that although we know we **possess** a body and a mind, for all practical purposes **we think that we are the body and the mind**? The simple logic to be applied to this: if we say, I have a body and a mind, the relationship between **my self** and the body and mind is one of **possessor and possessed**. The body and the mind are the objects possessed by the possessor, which is the real **I**. Why then, is this meaningless confusion between the possessor and the possessed? Do we not, in our practical life, always take the possessed for the possessor? Is not our ordinary consciousness of the **I** identical with the body and mind? Where has the possessor gone? In fact the real **I** is not recognized at all.

'... As soon as we realize the independent existence of that higher **I**, we enjoy the most intense degree of rest even in the midst of the most intense activity .

'... The philosophy behind the practice of relaxation is to experience by means of our meditation, the peaceful and all-perfect nature of the higher self. Its real nature has been very beautifully described in one of the *Upanishads*, by a very suggestive and deep simile, the tree of life.'

The Tree of Life

'**HUMAN LIFE** life has been compared to a gigantic tree which sends its roots deep down into the unfathomable bottom of the Unknown. It is nurtured and nourished by the sap of the unknown Infinite, which is Brahman. Its strong trunk is the trunk of karma, which has been attained, accumulated, through successions of incarnations. The whole tree is held firm by that trunk. In the shape of its different aptitudes and inclinations, it sends out many branches in every direction. These branches produce innumerable twigs, buds, leaves, flowers and fruit, representing the results of the impressions and experiences through which human life is advancing. The leaves appear in due time. They develop, attain maturity, remain on the tree for a while, and finally, having left their contribution to the upkeep of the tree, they drop off, making room for other leaves to come.

'In much the same way our experiences appear, remain for a while, mature and drop off. But when they drop off they do not vanish altogether. They leave their share of experience for the growth of the 'tree'. As in the case of the tree, so is human life. Flowers appear and gradually develop into fruit. Fruit in their maturity drop off, having left their contribution towards the development of the tree. The 'flowers and fruit' are the results of our actions; good, bad and indifferent. They appear, remain a while, and then drop off, contributing to the store-house of our **samskaras**[3].

'Seated at the top of the tree, but not supported by or depending upon it, is a Bird, self-poised, self-illumined and self-contained. It is always blissful, always cheerful. It never depends on anything for its existence, happiness or knowledge. It is radiating brilliance, effulgence; and the tree beneath is illumined by its heavenly light. This Bird never leaves its throne of glory at the top of the tree, for it has no desire, no wants. It has everything.

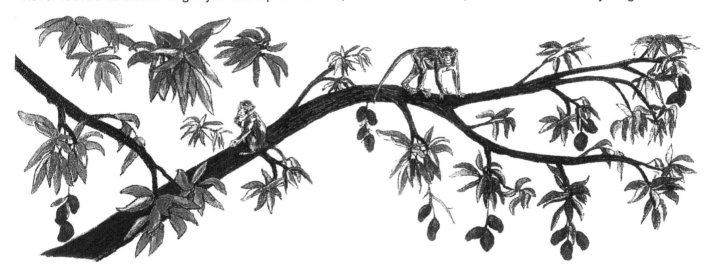

'There is another bird, very similar in appearance, which occupies the body of the tree. It has no fixed place of its own. It is moving constantly and hopping from branch to branch. It is always hungry and restless. Oh, the greed of this bird! The more it eats the more hungry it seems to be. Every moment is spent in finding and tasting new fruit. When it tastes a sweet one it experiences a temporary feeling of joy and happiness.

'But immediately that sense of satisfaction is gone, it is hungry again. It seizes another fruit which perhaps is bitter. Then it receives a shock and, looking around, it catches a glimpse of the beauty and radiance of the self-effulgent Bird above. It feels a great attraction and aspires to it. But, in the next moment, it forgets and darts after the fruit.

'While moving in search of the fruit the restless bird, being attracted unknowingly and imperceptibly by the other Bird, is slowly moving towards it in the form of a spiral. When a sense of satiety and satisfaction finally comes, the bird begins to feel disinclined to go round and search for the fruit. Sometimes it takes a direct flight towards the higher Bird and reaches it quickly. But more often the process of approach towards the higher one takes place rather slowly and gradually, until eventually, the lower bird comes very near the higher one, whose radiance and poise are reflected very distinctly in its personality. Finally it is absorbed into the upper Bird and loses its separate existence. It realizes that the lower bird is only a shadow of itself.

'All is **Maya**[3]. The only reality is the higher Bird, which took no active part in the process of the growth and development of the tree of life.

'Our real self is the higher Bird. The lower bird, or our physical and mental systems, is just the shadow of the higher one. The exercise of relaxation consists in putting oneself on the position of the top Bird.'

1. Translation: Juan Mascaro. The Upanishads. Penguin Classics; ISBN 0-14-044163-8
2. Meditation *by Monks of the Ramakrishna Order. ISBN 0-7025-0019-4*
3. Please refer to the Glossary.

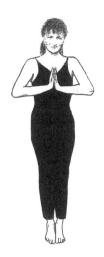

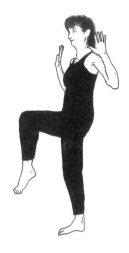

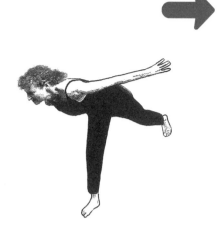

1. Stand with the hands in **Prayer**.

2. Shift your weight on to the right leg. **INHALE** as you raise your left knee. Bend your elbows and turn the palms to face forwards.

3. EXHALE as you swing your leg back and up and bring the hands back in **Flying Bird**, coming into the **Swallow**.

Introduction

THE BEGINNING of the sequence has an obvious breathing pattern but after **6** it is more obscure, and you may prefer to hold the postures for a few breaths.

It would be advantageous to practise the **Two Birds in a Tree** posture by itself before beginning the sequence. The hand mudras and the toes resting on the leg give it a delicate, ethereal quality. It will be more difficult to appreciate this within the sequence.

Birds Head Mudra is an unintentional mutation of mine. It transpired that the original mudra was **Bird of Paradise Mudra.** You can experiment and perhaps use **Birds Head** below and **Bird of Paradise** on top.

If you find the sequence too demanding, you can break it up into sections and do a few postures at a time. If you want to make it more demanding, you can repeat **2** and **3**, and **4** and **5,** at least twice, and trace the figure of eight in **9**, in both directions.

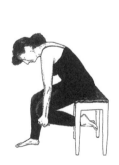

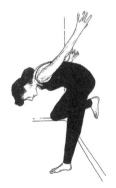

Two Birds in a Tree Variations

For those with limited mobility, this sequence can be practised sitting on a chair. It is best to use a chair without arms or obstructions under the seat. Similarly, it can be practised using a wall for support. Here are some examples of adaptations.

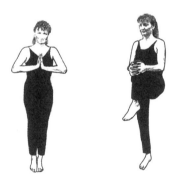

10. Return to **4** and hold for a few breaths before returning to **1**. *Change sides and repeat.*

*1. This posture is also called **Standing Wind Releasing Pose**.*
2. In her book Mudras, Yoga in the Hands *Gertrud Hirsch calls this **Mukula Mudra***, or **Beak Hand***.*
She says; **This energy-giving and relaxing mudra is placed on the organ or body part that hurts or feels tense. This is like directing a laser ray of regenerative energy to the respective body part or organ that needs healing.**

Weiser Books. ISBN 978-1-57863-139-1

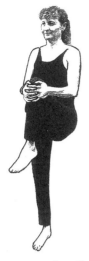

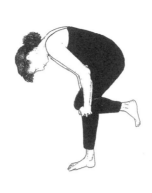

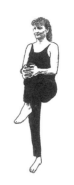

6. INHALE them up, returning to **4**.

5. EXHALE as you lower your knee and bring the foot behind.

4. INHALE as you swing the leg back to the front. Interlock the fingers round the knee and hug it close to you in the **Standing Knee Hug**[1]. Hold for a few breaths.

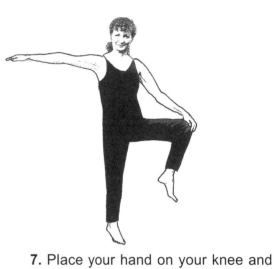

Two Birds in a Tree

7. Place your hand on your knee and move it out to the side. Stretch your right arm out to the right with the palm facing downwards. Hold for a few breaths, pushing your knee to the left and opening out the hip.

Bird's Head or Beak Hand Mudra

Bird of Paradise Mudra

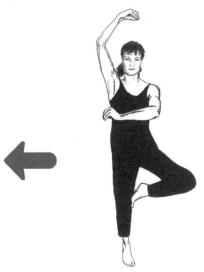

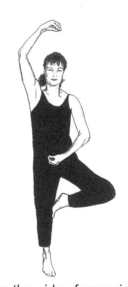

9. The **Higher Self,** your right hand, watches the **Lower Self** as it flies around. Make a figure of eight from side to side with your left hand, in either direction. *Repeat three times.*

8. Place your toes on the side of your right knee or thigh. Curve your right hand above your head and the left hand low with the fingers in **Bird's Head Mudra**[2]. This is **Two Birds in a Tree** pose.

You can either rest the ball of the foot on the knee, as illustrated, or the tips of your toes. You can lower the foot down the leg if you find the high position too difficult.

The Full Yogic Breath

I CONSIDER the **Full Yogic Breath** to be one of the most important things I have learnt in my life. Unfortunately I was not taught it until I did my Yoga Teachers Training Course at the age of 52. Meditation comes close behind in order of importance, because good breathing is a prerequisite to good meditation. High upper chest breathing, with lack of harmony between the diaphragm and the abdomen, will limit the development of your meditation.

Method

1. Lie on your back. The legs can be straight or slightly bent. Place your hands on the lower abdomen. Breathe with a completely relaxed abdomen. You will feel the abdomen rise on the **inhalation**, under the influence of the diaphragm, and flatten on the **exhalation** as the diaphragm contracts up into the rib cage. **Diaphragmatic breathing** brings air into the bottom part of your lungs.

2. Keep the left hand on the abdomen and place your right hand on the diaphragm. Direct your breath to the bottom of your lungs. Feel both hands rising and falling with the breath. *Repeat three times.*

3. Place your right hand half way up the right side of the rib cage. The thumb should be at the back and your fingers wrapped around the front of your ribs. **INHALE** into the middle part of your lungs. The ribs should move up and out to the sides on the **inhalation**, and lower on the **exhalation**. The abdomen will also rise and fall with the breath. *Repeat three times.*

4. Place your right hand on the upper chest and **INHALE** into the top part of the lungs. The right hand will rise as the sternum, ribs and area below the neck (the clavicles) lift up and out. The left hand on the abdomen will not rise as the diaphragm is passive. *Repeat three times.*

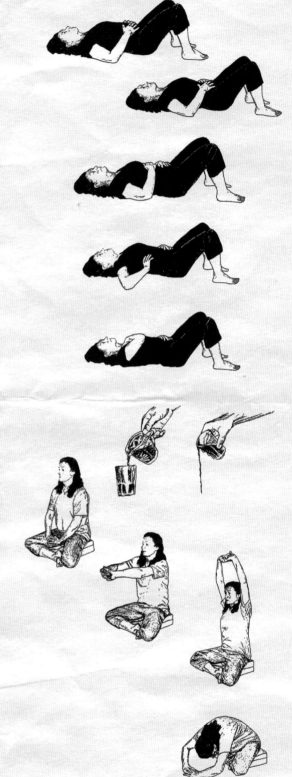

5. Now use all areas of the lungs; bottom, middle and top. This is the **Full Yogic Breath**. As you **INHALE**, fill the lungs from the bottom upwards, as if you were filling a glass of water. Both hands will rise. **EXHALE** from the top to the bottom, as if you were emptying a glass of water. Both hands will lower. *Repeat three times.*

6. Sit in **Easy Pose** with the legs lightly crossed, or in another comfortable sitting position. Interlock the fingers in **Venus Lock**. Lower your hands with the palms facing downwards. **EXHALE** completely and then **INHALE** into the bottom part of the lungs. Feel everything around the waist expand.

7. Continue to **INHALE** as you bring your arms up parallel to the floor, and breathe into the middle part of the lungs. Feel the ribs move up and out.

8. Raise your hands above your head and fill the top part of your lungs. Push away with the palms of your hands. This lifts the rib cage even further. Hold briefly.

9. To **EXHALE** reverse the procedure. Lower your hands slowly as you empty the lungs from top, middle to bottom. To completely empty the bottom part of the lungs, soften the elbows and lean forward and down. Use the abdominal muscles to squeeze the last bit of air out. **INHALE** the head up. Repeat from **6** to **9** three times.

The Hissing Breath

REST IN Extended Child's Pose with the hips on the heels and the hands stretched forwards. Use **Ujjayi** breathing to **INHALE** into the lower part of the lungs. As the diaphragm flattens and pushes the waist outwards, try to feel the back below the waist expanding.

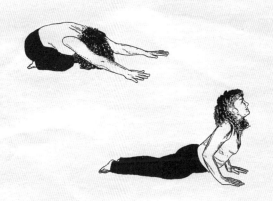

Hiss the **exhalation** out through your teeth as you swing forwards into the **Hissing Cobra**. You may need to move your hands forward a little.
INHALE back into **Extended Child's Pose**.
Repeat three times.

Figure of Eight Breathing

THE DIAGRAM uses a standing position as that makes it easier to demonstrate the **8**, but you will be lying on your back.

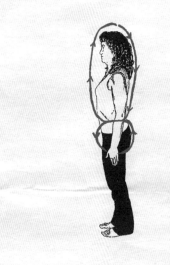

To visualize the **8**, bring your awareness to the base of the spine at the beginning of the **inhalation**. As you **INHALE** follow your awareness up the lower spine, through the waist, up the front of the body and face to the top of the head.

As you **EXHALE**, follow your awareness down the back of your head and neck, between the shoulder blades, down the back and through the waist. Follow it over the abdomen and through the legs to start the next **inhalation** at the base of the spine.

Your **inhalations** are the same length as your **exhalations**. *Continue for a few minutes.*

Now add the **Pelvic Rock**. As you **INHALE** press the lower spine into the floor. The tail bone will tilt up towards the ceiling.

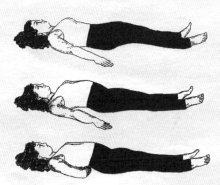

As you **EXHALE** the abdomen and spine arch upwards and the lower back comes off the floor. The tail bone tilts downwards.

The lower back should be high enough off the floor for you to place your forearm under the waist. This is only a guideline. Keep your hands by your sides, palms facing downwards.

When you combine the **8** and the **Pelvic Rock**, you will be pressing the lower spine into the floor as you **INHALE,** and arching the abdomen and spine up as you **EXHALE**. *Continue for a few minutes.*
When you feel ready, you can add a simple mantra of two syllables, for example; **Ha Sa**, **So Hum**, **Sat Nam** (**Sat** pronounced s<u>u</u>t as in b<u>u</u>t, **Nam** as in <u>arm</u>), or **Love** and **Peace**. Internalize (think) the first syllable on the **inhalation** and the second on the **exhalation**.

Here are some different meanings given to these mantras:
Ha means **Shiva** or **Sun**. **Sa** means **Shakti** or **Moon**. **So Hum** means **I am that** or **I am that I am**.
Sat means **Truth**. **Nam** means **Identity**. There are many different interpretations when you put the two together, such as: *Truth is my identity*, or *The essence of God is within me*, or *I bow to the truth*.

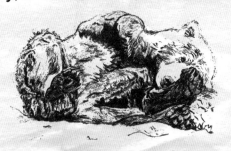

The Nose or Sniff Breath

THIS IS an upper chest breath. The nose is used like a suction pump to bring a large amount of air into the lungs quickly. The nostrils are likely to be sucked towards each other. There is minimal diaphragm awareness. The rib cage should move up and out on the inhalation and lower on the exhalation.

The Sniffing Breath

THIS IS is a particularly good exercise for anybody with an immobile rib cage. I find some of my yoga pupils, especially those who are asthma sufferers, have very limited expansion of the rib cage when they start coming to classes. If they inhale with their hands on the rib cage, as illustrated, their ribs do not move up and out. Some elderly people have used restricted breathing all their lives and they are completely unaware of it. However, I find that once my pupils are aware of a problem and they consciously work on expanding the rib cage, there can be an improvement within three to four months.

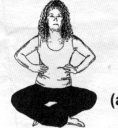

Sit in any position that allows you to concentrate on the upper part of the body. Place your hands on the lower rib cage with the thumbs at the back. EXHALE completely, as in (a). Be aware of the lowered rib cage.

(a)

First, aim to fill the lungs in three sniffs. Partially fill the lungs with the first sniff and then pause (hold the ribs and diaphragm still) for a few seconds. Take another sniff and fill up a bit more and pause again. On the third sniff try to fill the lungs completely, as in (b), and then pause for about 10 seconds before exhaling slowly.

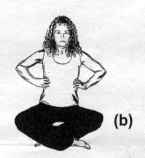

(b)

Keep the mouth closed throughout. Feel your hands move up and out with each sniff. The shoulders and clavicles (area under the neck) will expand outwards and rise automatically, but try to make the movement of the ribs feel independent from the shoulders. The shoulders do not have to move upwards when the rib cage expands. Breathing is more efficient if the shoulders have minimal upward movement.
Repeat as many times as you feel you need to.

Variation 1
Proceed as above, but this time, take six little sniffs to fill the lungs completely. Pause for a little longer and then slowly EXHALE. *Repeat as above.*

Variation 2
This variation uses the mantra Sa Ta Na Ma. This translates as; **Infinity, Life, Death** and **Rebirth**. It is best to sing the mantra a few times before internalising it.

INHALE taking four sniffs and think one syllable per sniff. EXHALE the same way, lowering the rib cage with four separate little exhalations and thinking, singing or saying Sa Ta Na Ma.
Repeat as above.

The Whistling Breath

The whistle can be voiced or unvoiced; i.e. you may whistle a note or just hear the noise of the breath pushing through the lips. You may sit in any position that allows you to lower the top part of the body forwards. Here we are using cushions.

Place your hands on the upper thighs with the palms facing downwards. INHALE into the bottom part of the lungs using Ujjayi breathing. Be aware of the expansion around the waist and the lower and upper back. For the exhalation make a small hole in the lips by tensing them forwards. You can use the lips as a valve to stop the air from coming out too quickly. This will slow down the exhalation.

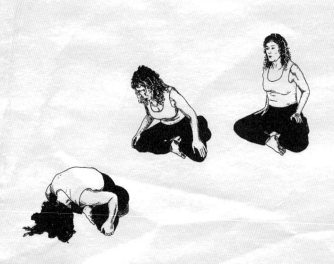

Slide the hands down the thighs as you lower the head towards the floor and whistle the breath out through the lips. Use the abdominal muscles to push the last bit of air out of the lungs. INHALE the head up. *Repeat three times.*

You can also hum a note in the same way. There will be a tiny space between the lips for the breath to pass through. You can experiment with low, middle and high notes.

Square Breathing

Method

Lie on your back. Breathe with a completely relaxed abdomen. You can place your hands on the lower abdomen and feel it rise when you INHALE and fall when you EXHALE. Breathe in four equal parts. Start off counting in **4**s.

After about four breaths, increase your counting to **6**s and then **8**s. Continue to increase your counting but always stay within your comfort zone. If you reach **15** you will be breathing one breath per minute.

INHALE   Pause

EXHALE   Pause

INHALE for 4 seconds

Pause for 4 seconds

Pause for 4 seconds

EXHALE for 4 seconds

Breaths per minute

Method

In this practice **exhalations** are twice as long as **inhalations**. Start with an **inhalation** of **four** seconds and an **exhalation** of **eight** seconds. In the calculation below, I have suggested how many breaths you make for each counting. You can make more repetitions if you feel you are still within your comfort zone. The quality of the **inhalation** usually determines the quality of the **exhalation**. If your **inhalations** are weak, work on the **Sniffing Breath** and the **Dynamic Breath** to increase the expansion of the rib cage.

4 and 8 = 5 times a minute. Continue for between 5 and 7 breaths.
6 and 12 = about 3 times a minute. Continue for 4 breaths.
8 and 16 = 2½ times a minute. 3 breaths.
10 and 20 = twice a minute. 2 breaths.
20 and 40 = once a minute. 1 breath.

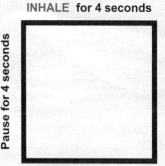

Wave Breathing

It helps to visualize the breath like a wave. The crest (the **inhalation**) happens after a build up of energy and it is powerful. The trough (the **exhalation**) goes on for a long time until the next build up of energy resolves into another crest. In practice you can make your **inhalations** dynamic and your **exhalations** a natural, peaceful resolution of that energy. You can pause for a long time before you **inhale** again. There is still plenty of oxygen in your lungs.

You can use the mantra **Om Ah Hum** as you practise **Wave Breathing**. Say the mantra out loud a few times and then internalize it. Think **Om** as you **inhale** and **Ah** as you go over the top of your **inhalation** (like the crest of a wave). Think **Hum** as you **exhale**. The pause at the end of the **exhalation** is very special. It is a natural empty space where your thinking stops and your mind goes blank. Just enjoy the unusual sensation.

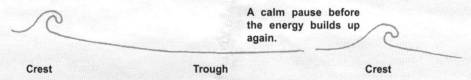

A calm pause before the energy builds up again.

Crest   Trough   Crest

The Dynamic Breath

Method

When you practise the **Sniffing Breath** you are expanding the rib cage in stages. In **The Dynamic Breath** you expand it to full capacity quickly. Sit or stand with your head aligned over the pelvic floor. Open the armpits to allow the rib cage to expand.

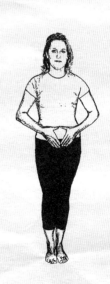

Exhale and then **inhale**, with a powerful breath, and fill the lungs completely from the bottom to the top. Pause for a few seconds and then **exhale** through the mouth making a loud Zzzzzzzz sound. Continue the slow exhalation until you have pushed the last bit of air from the bottom of the lungs with the abdominal muscles.

Now you are ready to take your first **Dynamic Breath**. It is a very powerful movement. The diaphragm and rib cage experience their complete range of movement, from maximum contraction to maximum expansion, in about three seconds. The breath will be noisy and the sides of the nose may be sucked inwards. Pause briefly and then repeat the **exhalation** as described above.

When you have practised it a few times, place your hands on the upper abdomen with the thumbs and first fingers touching. Continue and observe the hands moving outwards on the **inhalation** and backwards, slowly towards the spine, on the **exhalations**. To help monitor your progress, and increase your concentration, try counting on your **exhalations**.

The Bandhas

THE BODY has an electrical circuit. Electricity needs effective regulation and control; e.g. fuses and switches. The ancient Yogis, some of whom spent many hours every day directing energy round their bodies, developed an equivalent regulatory system. The **Bandhas** are used to prevent damage to the nervous system and electrical or pranic short-circuiting in the body. **Bandha** means **lock**. The system should be taught by an experienced teacher in an appropriate environment. It is beyond the scope of this book. This page is a brief introduction in preparation for the **Four Directions**.

The Three Bandhas: Mula Bandha comes from the Sanskrit word **mula** which means **root**. It refers to the muscles in between the legs called the **pelvic floor** or **perineum**. Uddiyana Bandha comes from **ut** or **di** meaning **to fly up**. There are contrasting definitions but it involves the abdomen and diaphragm and is often called the **Stomach Lock**. Jalandhara Bandha comes from **jala** which means **net** or **network** (the network of nerves and arteries in the neck) and **dhara** which means **pulling upwards**. It is often called the **Chin Lock**.

A simplified version of Uddiyanna Bandha followed by Maha Bandha (applying the three locks)

1. Stand in **Horse Riding Stance** with the hands pushing down on the knees. **EXHALE** completely by flattening the abdomen, pushing the air from the bottom of the lungs, and lowering the rib cage to push the air from the top of the lungs.

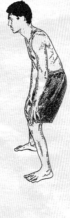

3. Return to **2.**

2. Take a **Full Yogic Breath** (bottom, middle and top of the lungs) and expand the rib cage as much as you can. Now keep the rib cage fully extended but flatten the abdomen and contract the diaphragm. This will push the air from the bottom part of the lungs.

The diaphragm can be moved right up into the rib cage, like an upturned cereal bowl. This action stretches the diaphragm, and the internal organs will be pushed in and up. This gives a beneficial massage to the colon and large and small intestines.

When you feel ready, hold the posture, with maximum contraction of the abdomen and diaphragm, for 20 seconds. Then slowly release them and breathe normally.
Repeat two or three times.

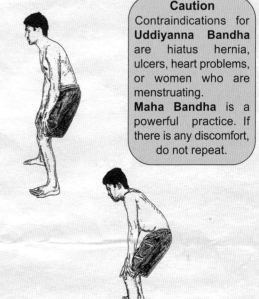

> **Caution**
> Contraindications for **Uddiyanna Bandha** are hiatus hernia, ulcers, heart problems, or women who are menstruating.
> **Maha Bandha** is a powerful practice. If there is any discomfort, do not repeat.

After establishing **Uddiyana Bandha**, apply **Mula Bandha** by tensing the muscles of the pelvic floor and pulling them in and up. Now apply **Jalandhara Bandha** by either tucking in the chin or pulling the chin backwards. Both stretch the back of the neck and contract the throat area. Hold as above.

To come out of **Maha Bandha**, release the **pelvic floor** first and then the **stomach** and **throat** locks. **INHALE** and breathe normally. It is important to follow this procedure.

Yoga Nidra

This is usually translated as **Yogic Sleep** (**nidra** means **sleep**). It is the ancient tantric practice of **Nyasa** (this means **to take the mind to a point**). Swami Satyananda Sariswati revived the practice while he was living in Swami Sivananda's Ashram in Rishikesh, in about 1940[1]. It is now frequently practised at the end of yoga classes, but it has proved so beneficial that it is also used in other healing situations; e.g. to relieve post traumatic stress disorders and to remove negative behaviour patterns.

In Yoga Nidra the mind is suspended between wakefulness and sleep for usually between 10 or 15 minutes. Unlike meditation, it requires an external ingredient. This will either be a person talking or an audio presentation, e.g. a tape or CD. The spoken word keeps the mind awake by skillfully moving it from one point to another, either by systematically moving awareness round the body (as in **Gold Yoga Nidra**) or through visualization (as in **Tropical Island Yoga Nidra**).

Concentration, unlike meditation, is not necessary. The spoken word, delivered with sensitivity and at an appropriate speed, will create the necessary awareness to keep the mind awake while the body hovers near a state of sleep. Unlike meditation, it is nearly always practised lying on the back, with the palms facing upwards and the feet falling apart naturally. It can be practised sitting on a chair if lying on the back is uncomfortable.

In **Yoga Nidra** we relax the mind by first relaxing the body. In meditation we stabilize the body and then direct our energies through our chosen point, or points, of concentration. In both methods there are profound benefits to the body which have all been scientifically proven. However, both also work at a much deeper level.

In **Yoga Nidra** the barriers between the conscious, unconscious and subconscious minds dissolve. Some teachers liken this to **the opening of the third eye**[2]. It certainly facilitates the use of our intuition and psychic abilities. It is like opening a door to another world, as many artists and scientists have discovered.

➡

THIS COMES from a workshop given by Alex Boyd at the BWY London Region Festival, 2008. He says of 'The Four Directional' exercise: *It is a Daoyin (respiration therapy), predominantly breathing exercise but also involves Yijin (dynamic tension), Qigong (energy work) and Visualization. It is done slowly with the hands mainly closed off to help nourish Qi (energy). The exercise is part of 'Lishi', as taught by the International Daoist Society.*

I have linked it with the **Bandhas** because you will find yourself applying **Uddiyana Bandha** and **Mula Bandha** during this practice. Before lifting or pushing anything, most people will automatically tense the pelvic floor and contract the abdominal muscles.

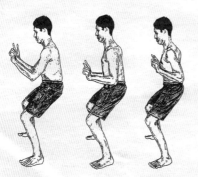

Visualization

Imagine you are pushing a very heavy pile of boxes in different directions.

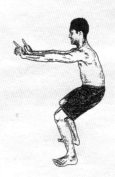

1. Position yourself in **Horse Riding** stance. Lift the hands and close the middle, ring and little fingers into the palms of your hands.
Leave the index finger extended.
The thumbs stay on the outside and follow the direction of the pushing.
On the inhalation, circle the hands inwards by lowering them down and back.

2. EXHALE slowly through the mouth on the letter S, making a hissing sound as you direct your hands to those imaginary boxes and forcefully push them away.
As you direct the energy into your arms, you will feel the dynamic tension there. Become aware of the way the rest of your body is responding.
Repeat three times.
At the end of the last long exhalation release the tension and prepare for the next direction.

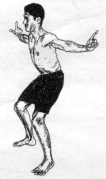

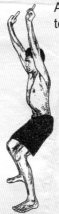

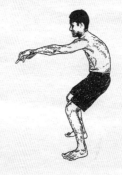

3. Repeat the procedure, circling the hands to the sides and pushing away a pile of boxes on each side.

4. Now imagine you are pushing a pile of boxes up onto a shelf. In this posture the rib-cage will be lifted further, giving more scope for the diaphragm to move upwards.

5. Repeat the procedure pushing the boxes downwards.

Yoga Nidra (continued)

During complete relaxation, our consciousness effortlessly shifts away from our intellectually imposed structures. These become rather like a mental prison. We all construct complicated ways of perceiving ourselves and defining ourselves. These can be based on misconceptions. They can hold us back and reinforce negative behaviour. When we are released from such constraints, we are more receptive to a lot of things, including suggestion. For this reason, some teachers of **Yoga Nidra** use **Sankalpas**[3] (a resolution). At the beginning and end of the practice, positive seeds are skillfully planted into the receptive mind.

Some teachers claim that no personality is beyond reformation through **Yoga Nidra**. Taking into consideration the fact that the beneficiary just has to lie on their back and make no effort, it is a unique tool for transformation. The spoken word is the transforming energy. Never come out of Yoga Nidra quickly. Carefully and slowly readjust to the outside world after deep relaxation.

---

1. *Swami Satyananda Saraswati founded the Bihar School of Yoga in 1964. His book* Yoga Nidra *was published by Yoga Publications Trust in 1976. ISBN 81-85787-12-3*
2. *This is often said to correspond to the pineal gland which secretes chemicals that have a calming effect on the body and expand the activities of the mind.*
3. *Here are three examples of Sankalpas: Day by Day my heart is becoming lighter and brighter and warmer and kinder; I am becoming a healing channel for Universal Love; I choose to direct my attention towards things that make me healthy, happy and contented.*

Gold Yoga Nidra

THIS IS a basic yoga Nidra, working round the body and dwelling on each area for a short time. This takes you on a corresponding journey round the sensory motor strip of the brain. This has the effect of completely relaxing these areas as you pass through them.

I do not like to use the word 'relax' too much in my lessons. Some people get anxious when they are asked to relax, and it has the opposite effect. When you suggest to people that they feel heavy, they automatically seem to relax and it is more productive.

Method

Lie on your back with your eyes closed and the palms of your hands facing upwards. Bend your knees if you need to. Breathe with a completely relaxed abdomen.

Visualize a soft, light gold. This colour is sometimes called white gold. It is a more relaxing colour than energizing bright gold. As the body parts or areas are mentioned, **INHALE** this gentle colour into them. Feel as if they are expanding with light gold.

Bring your awareness to your big toes. **INHALE** and breathe gold into your big toes. **EXHALE** slowly and visualize your big toes shining with gold. Now connect to your second toe, third toe, fourth toe and the little toe. **INHALE** and breathe this calming gold into all your toes. **EXHALE** and visualize the toes glowing with gold.

Now take your awareness to the soles of your feet. **INHALE** and feel as if you are filling the soles of your feet with this beautiful colour. **EXHALE** and feel your soles expanding with gold.

Repeat the procedure passing through the heels, ankles and the top of your feet. Continue up to the lower legs and calves, the knees (top of the knees and the bottom of the knees) and thighs (top of the thighs and bottom of the thighs).

Now take your awareness up into the abdomen. Breathe this soft, gentle, light gold into the abdomen. Let the internal organs feel very heavy and very sleepy ... very heavy and very sleepy. Feel the buttocks pressing heavily into the floor ... sinking further and further into the floor ... and the legs and feet getting heavier and heavier and sleepier and sleepier. Take your awareness up the lower back, through the diaphragm and into the lungs and the chest. As you **INHALE** completely fill the lungs from the bottom to the top with this beautiful gold.

Bring your awareness to both thumbs. Repeat the procedure, breathing into the thumbs first, and then into the first fingers, second fingers, third fingers and little fingers. Then take your awareness to the palms of your hands. Breathe the gold into the palms of your hands and then ... let the palms of your hands feel very heavy and very sleepy ... let both your hands feel very heavy and very sleepy.

Now take your awareness up the wrists, lower arms, elbows and upper arms. Breathe the gold into them. Then move on to the armpits and shoulders. Breathe the gold into them and then ... feel the heaviness of the top part of your body on the floor and your shoulders and shoulder blades pressing down into the floor ... sinking further and further into the floor ... and your arms and your hands feeling heavier and heavier and sleepier and sleepier.

Take your awareness to the point between the shoulder blades and then up the back of your neck. **INHALE** as you wrap the gentle gold round the sides of your neck and up under your chin. Bring your awareness into the jaw, lips, cheeks, nose, eyes, eyebrows and forehead. Slowly breathe soft, light gold into all these areas ... Feel the top lip resting gently on the bottom lip and the top eyelid gently touching the bottom eyelid.

Now breathe the gold up from your lungs, through the hollow spaces of your neck, to the back of your throat. Breathe the gold into the back of your throat and your tongue ... Take your awareness up the back of your nose, into the nostrils and the sinuses (hollow spaces in the front of your face). Take it to the hollow spaces behind your eyes and the hollow spaces in your brain. Now breathe this gentle, calming gold into all these areas.

Take your awareness to the back of your head and find the place that is touching the floor. As you **INHALE** feel as if your head is like a golden sculpture. Feel it getting heavier and heavier and sinking further and further into the floor.

Finally breathe this lovely gold into the whole of your mind and brain. Let your mind go completely blank. Get rid of all the words in your mind ... no words ... just feel the gold gently caressing all of your body and mind.

Return to normal awareness very slowly.

Observations

You can vary this simple yoga Nidra by changing the colours. When it is spring you can use daffodil yellow. In the autumn you can use warm colours; golds, reds and browns. You can breathe sunlight, a bright radiant energy, into the body in the same way.

Tropical Island Yoga Nidra

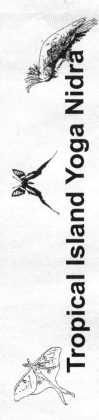

THE INSPIRATION for the following visualizations in **Tropical Island Yoga Nidra** came from *Yoga Education for Children*[1], which I have modified, adapted and use for adults.

I have added detail and suggested bending the knees, to imitate mountain ranges, and turning the palms downwards. Some teachers of Yoga Nidra would say that these suggestions would interfere with the relaxation process, and that it should always be practised with the palms facing upwards and the legs straight. I have not removed them as my pupils have benefited from the practice as it is presented here and I feel it would diminish the experience.

Method

Lie on a blanket or mat, and make sure your body is sufficiently comfortable for you to remain still and peaceful for at least ten minutes.

Imagine your body is a tropical island in the middle of the Pacific Ocean. The island rises sharply from the deep sea bed. It is large enough to have a range of mountains. The mountains are your knees and they are high enough to reach way up into the clouds and there is snow on top.

The sky is very clear and blue. The sun is shining brightly overhead and it is very hot, but there is a gentle breeze coming in from the sea. Imagine the sea lapping round the edge of your body. Visualize the gentle waves breaking on the sandy beaches.

Let's think about the river systems on the island. Rivers run down from the mountains on every side. Some run over your feet to the sea and some run down onto the grassy plains that cover the abdomen. Other little rivers and streams come down from your forehead, and trickle over the rolling hills to the grassy plains. Others run down the arms from the shoulders and join the sea in the rocky coves in-between the fingers. This is where the people who live on the island keep their fishing boats.

Tropical forests grow up the sides of the mountains until the terrain gets too rocky and rugged. There are lots of fruit trees on the island. Coconuts grow by the beaches and there are mango and papaya trees, bananas and lychees and many more. Creepers with large leaves twist up the trees and there are beautiful orchids and flowers.

Lots of birds and monkeys live in the trees. There are large red and blue macaws, birds of paradise, parakeets of every colour, yellow canaries, and in the mountains there are golden eagles. There are big and little monkeys, and there are two families of gorillas on the island. They sometimes come down onto the grassy plains.

Tigers and leopards also live in the forest, and on the ground you find lots of deer and wild boar. There are a few herds of elephants.

Now the afternoon sun is making a little monkey sleepy and it curls up on your forehead and goes to sleep. A large, bright yellow butterfly flutters down and lands on your nose. A large, bright blue butterfly lands on each of your big toes.

There are small villages all over the island. The indigenous people live as their ancestors have lived for many generations. There is a village on each shoulder, and one on the back of each hand near the harbours. There is one on top of each foot, and more on the river banks.

The islanders live a simple life. They have everything they need and live harmoniously. They build their own huts and houses out of wood and leaves. Some of them have returned from a fishing trip in the sea and they are preparing a fire for the early evening meal. As the sun is starting to set, they all gather round, men, women and children, and share out the hot fish and other tropical delights. They use banana leaves as plates.

The large sun is starting to go down over the edge of the sea. It is dark orange and red, with the surrounding sky glowing with streaks of pink, purple, orange and yellow. This reflects onto the sea, and from the island, it all looks like a big ball of fire.

A white dove has been flying across the ocean from Australia and is feeling tired. As the sun disappears over the horizon, it lands on the Heart Centre, in the middle of the chest, and puts its head under its wing. Soon it drifts off into deep sleep. As darkness descends the stars shine brightly. You can see the Milky Way stretched out across the night sky. The nocturnal birds and animals come out of their nests whilst the other creatures slowly curl up and go to sleep.

Let us stay with the island a little longer and just feel its gentle vibrations, and drink in the beauty of nature ...

Pause for as long as you want to.

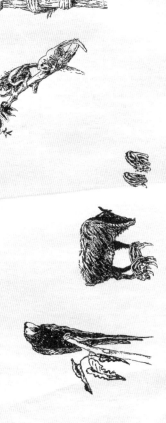
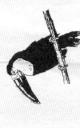
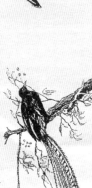

1. Yoga Education for Children *by Satyananda Paramahansa, published by the International Yoga Fellowship Movement, 1985. ISBN 81-85787-38-7*

Self Healing Meditation
The Mind Medicine Room

THE INSPIRATION for this meditation comes from **Mind Magic** by Betty Shine[1]. I have used it many times at the end of yoga classes, during relaxation. It has evolved over the years. I have added detail but the essence remains. I have written it here as if I were saying it in a class.

Method

Lie on your back or sit on a chair, with your eyes closed. Take a few breaths with a completely relaxed abdomen. Try to exaggerate everything I ask you to visualize. When I ask you to imagine you are walking down a corridor, make it a mass of swirling colours or a wood panelled corridor with portraits on the walls. Really go 'over the top' with everything I ask you to visualize.

Imagine you are walking down a corridor. At the end of the corridor, there is a door, and your name is written on the door in very beautiful writing … There is a key in the door. Make it the kind of key you would find in *Alice in Wonderland*, a very eccentric key … Unlock the door and take the key out. Go through the door, close it, and lock it from the inside.

Look around. You will find yourself in your self-healing, mind medicine room. It is a large room with two large windows at the far end … Let's put a carpet on the floor … Visualize a really luxurious, extravagant carpet … Now wander over your carpet to the windows … Put some curtains around the windows, very special curtains.

The windows are overlooking parkland, so there is a lot of grass, many trees, and a lake in the distance. Visualize all the animals; the horses, cows, sheep and deer.

Now turn round and look around your room. You will notice some furniture. There is a chair. It is a very special chair. It is your self healing chair, so imagine what it looks like, the shape, colours and textures … Now go and sit down on your self-healing chair and think of all the things you would like to heal. They can be mental, emotional or physical, anything you are not too happy about.

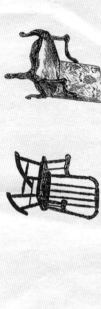

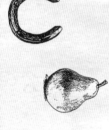

When you are ready, look around the room. You will notice some shelves on a wall. There are jam jars on the shelves and the jam jars have labels on them. Let's wander over to the shelves. Take off a jam jar. You will see a pen. Pick up the pen and write on the label the first thing you would like to heal … Put down the pen and imagine the kind of pill, potion or remedy that would cure this particular problem. It doesn't have to be a conventional pill. It can be a chocolate teddy bear, a marzipan apple or a purple jewel. Really go over the top …

Now take the lid off the jam jar and put it down … Put your hand inside the jam jar and take out one or two of these very special pills and swallow them … Put the lid back on the jam jar and put it back on the shelf.

We'll repeat the procedure. You are a very lucky person if you only have one problem. Take another jam jar off the shelf, pick up the pen and continue as above …

When you are ready, wander back to your self-healing chair. Sit down on it and imagine all the shapes and colours being absorbed by your mind and body …

Now walk over to the door, unlock it and take the key out. Go through the door, close it and lock it from the outside and wander off back down your corridor …

You can return to your self-healing mind medicine room any time you want to and build up your own magic pharmacy of special remedies and potions.

Observations

This is a very powerful meditation. You are opening a door in the right side of your brain and making a suggestion. Little by little you will find a different way of coping with a situation or an answer to a problem. It works in a very subtle way. Some times you don't notice the changes that are happening, until one day, you realize that the problem has gone away.

Some people can't visualize. When I did this meditation at Inglewood Health Hydro, a lady came up at the end of the lesson and said it was the first time she had been able to visualize in her life, so persevere. Try drawing a picture of a magic remedy that would help you to visualize and put it in a special box and … just wait.

1. Mind Magic by Betty Shine, a Corgi Book, ISBN 0-552-13671-9
Betty Shine is best known as a clairvoyant and healer. She was also a yoga teacher. She passed over in 2002. Before she died, she asked her daughter Janet to carry on her good work. Janet Shine is also a yoga teacher.

Some ideas for your magic pharmacy

Standing Pratyahara

THE INSPIRATION behind **Standing Pratyahara** came from a workshop by Rupert Linton at the BWY London Region Festival in 2008. Rupert says that the influences that helped him develop this idea came from Rolfing, Donna Farhi, Andrea Olsen and Rosie Spiegel.

Think of withdrawing the senses from the outside world in the same way that a tortoise brings in its legs and arms under its shell. It keeps them there until it needs to move again. For best results, keep the eyes closed. If you start to feel dizzy it is best to avoid this practice. Do not attempt to interfere with the breath in any way. Occasionally be a witness and have a peep at what it is doing.

Moving in a **Figure of Eight** is a variation. The central point you establish will be the middle of the figure of eight.

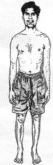 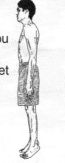 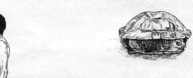

1. Stand with the feet slightly apart and the hands by your sides. The feet should be facing forwards. The eyes look straight ahead.

2. INHALE as you go up on tiptoes. **EXHALE** the feet down. *Repeat three times.*

   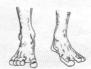 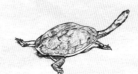 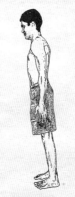

3. Lift the toes and spread them out wide. Lower the little toes first and then lower the others. Keep them as wide apart as you can.

4. Try lifting the three middle toes by themselves. This improves with practise.

5. Without changing the alignment of the spine, dig in with the toes and tilt the body forward in the **Forward Tilt**. Do not expect to tilt very far. *Repeat three times.* On the third tilt, let the heels come very slightly off the floor.

6. Establish a central point in the middle of your feet. Align the head and spine comfortably over this central point. Now start to make a small circle clockwise around this central point.
Increase the size of the circle until you feel your weight shifting from the front to the sides and backs of your feet.
Continue to circle round about eight times or until you start to feel calm and peaceful.

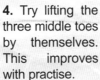 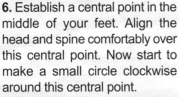 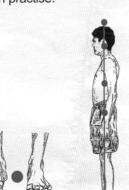 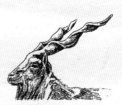

The handsome horns of the Markhor, a wild goat from Afghanistan, demonstrate one of natures ingenious spiral creations.

7. When you are ready, shift your awareness to the centre of the abdomen. Locate a point and align it directly above the lower central point. Start to circle round again in the same direction.

8. When you feel the time is right, shift your awareness to the **Heart Centre**. Find a similar point in the middle of the chest and align it over the other central points. Start to circle round again. The circle may become a little smaller.

9. When you are ready shift your awareness to the **Throat Centre**. You can choose a point in the middle of the throat or you can place your tongue on the roof of the mouth. Continue to circle round with a slightly smaller circle.
After about eight circles, pause and become aware of the smells you are experiencing and then the taste in your mouth. Be aware of your skin covering your entire body. Feel your skin touching between your fingers. Feel your clothes touching your skin and your skin touching your clothes.

10. When you are ready, take your awareness to the top of your head. Start to circle round again. Make the circle about the size of a grapefruit. Slowly reduce the size of the circle in stages, to the size of an orange, then an apple, plum, grape and finally to then size of a pin head.
Take about a minute to stop moving and reconnect to the outside world. Listen to the noises you can hear and very slowly open your eyes. Do not hurry the reconnection phase. Take as long as you need to and slowly merge again with your surroundings.

Nose and Throat Breathing

THIS SECTION is inspired by Sophie Gabriel's book *Breathe for Life*[1]. She is not a Yoga teacher but she is familiar with yogic breathing and praises its effectiveness. She teaches correct breathing techniques from the perspective of personal well-being.

She uses the concept of **Nose and Throat Breathing**. This input led me to make the connection between **Nose Breathing** and the **Sympathetic Nervous System**, and **Throat Breathing** and the **Parasympathetic Nervous System**.

In **Nose Breathing** the sensations are felt in the nose. In **Throat Breathing** they are felt in the throat.

Throat Breathing
or Ujjayi in Yoga
and Ibuki in Karate

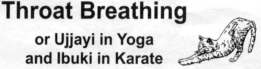

I WILL start with some quotes from Sophie Gabriel's book:

Throat breathing is the kind of breathing that happens naturally when good quality deep breathing occurs ... The sound also gives you the opportunity to monitor and observe the quality and duration of your breathing.

When I am teaching someone how to breathe a good quality breath, the first concept I teach is how to throat breath, and I do not continue with the rest of the training until they have grasped it.

Other names for **Ujjayi** are Victorious Breath[2], Ocean Sounding Breath, Psychic Breath (because of its effect on the mind) and I have even heard it called Darth Vader Breath. I have also added Steam Engine Breath and Dozy Dog Breath (after observing that my brother's dog Rolo, a chocolate Labrador, is an excellent ujjayi breather when he is very relaxed).

Although most people do ujjayi naturally when they are sleeping, or concentrating and relaxing deeply, I find that some of my pupils are timid, awkward ujjayi breathers and don't adjust well to producing the sound in class. In contrast some pupils find it so easy and beneficial that they tend to do it to some degree (loudly or softly) for most of the lesson.

I personally find it so beneficial that I make a point of doing it most of the day (you can do it silently but still put the emphasis on the throat) as a way of inducing the parasympathetic nervous system and saving energy.

You sometimes hear of high achievers who only need a few hours sleep a night. There was an obituary in *The Week* magazine (3 November 07) for the spiritual guru Sri Chinmoy. He claimed only to have needed 90 minutes of sleep a night.

As well as being very strong, Chinmoy was extraordinarily prolific, said The Times. Over the course of his life, he is said to have written 1,500 books, 115,000 poems, and 20,000 songs and to have painted an astonishing 200,000 paintings.

Chinmoy entered very deep states of meditation and taught ujjayi breathing to his pupils. His breathing is most likely to have been of a parasympathetic nature most of the time.

Here are some quotes about ujjayi from the *Hatha Yoga Pradipika*[3].

The practice of ujjayi is so simple that it can be done in any position and anywhere ... It helps relax the physical body and the mind, and develops awareness of the subtle body and psychic sensitivity. Ujjayi promotes internalization of the senses and pratyahara[4].

Ujjayi is especially recommended for people who have insomnia and mental tension. It is a must in the yogic management of heart disease. However, anyone with low blood pressure must first correct their condition before taking up the practice.

Method

The original method was making the noise in the throat while inhaling through both nostrils, retaining the breath and then exhaling quietly and slowly through the left nostril. These are slightly simplified quotes from the same version of the *Hatha Yoga Pradipika*.

Closing the mouth, draw in the breath through both nostrils till the breath fills the space from the throat to the heart with the noise. Perform kumbhaka (pause and hold the breath) *and exhale through the left nostril ...*
This is called ujjayi and it can be done while moving, standing, sitting or walking.

During the last century, some yoga teachers discovered the benefits of using ujjayi during sequential posture work. They omitted the pause and made the noise on inhalation and exhalation. This is now the accepted practice in some yoga classes.

The noise is made by gently constricting the opening of the throat and creating some resistance to the passage of air. It cannot be made without engaging the diaphragm. The diaphragm expands downwards to draw the air in through the slightly closed throat.

Some teachers think it causes tension in the throat and avoid it, but if it is done gently, using our natural technique, it should have the opposite effect.

1. Breathe for Life, *Basic Health Publications, Inc. ISBN 1-59120-002-4*
2. **Ujji** is the root which means 'to conquer' or 'acquire by contest'.
3. *From the Hatha Yoga Pradipika. Commentary by Swami Muktibodhananda Saraswati, under guidance of Swami Satyananda Saraswati. Bihar School of Yoga. No ISBN.*
4. *The fifth stage in Patanjali's Eight Limbs of Raja Yoga.*
It is the process of disconnecting from the outside world and taking the senses inwards before concentration and meditation.

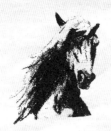

The Sympathetic and Parasympathetic Nervous Systems

THE NETWORK of nerves that connect to the spinal cord and brain (the Peripheral Nervous System) has two overlapping parts. They are the somatic (under conscious control) and autonomic (self-regulating).

The **Autonomic Nervous System** normally functions outside conscious, willed control[1]; e.g. regulating breathing, digestion and pupil dilation. It has two counteracting parts, the **Sympathetic** and **Parasympathetic**.

Sympathetic

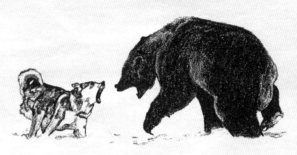

Bodily functions speed up.

There is a high consumption of energy with some wastage of energy.

It operates when we are in **Survival Mode**[2]. This is the **Fight or Flight** response. In a frightening, life-threatening situation we have to react quickly by either attacking the threat or running away. This can be a sudden, dramatic happening or a continual sense of unease[3].

The system speeds up the heartbeat, sends more blood to the relevant muscles and enlarges the pupils of the eye to enable it to use all available light. It takes blood away from the digestive tract and sends it to the parts that need to react to the emergency. Feeding and reproduction can be part of the survival mode.

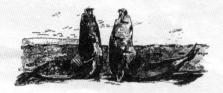

Body Language

Movements speed up. There is an emphasis of movement in the hands, nose and face. In extreme cases there will be quick upper chest **Nose Breathing**.

The obvious example is the backward ears and flared nostrils of a horse when it is angry, frightened or threatened. One of my pupils says her husband flares his nostrils when he is angry.

This newspaper headline describes a woman defending herself in debate. ***Nostrils flaring, face flushed, she snapped: He's just wrong***[4].

Parasympathetic

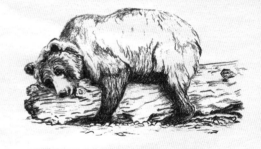

Bodily functions slow down.

There is a low consumption of energy with some storage of energy.

It operates when we are secure, confident and contented.

The **Four Rs** are usually used to describe its activities:
Rest, Relax, Restore and **Renew**.

The heart slows down and the digestive system is well supplied with blood. The pupils contract as orientation turns inwards, away from external things.

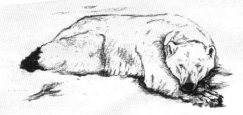

Body Language

Movements slow down.

The hands and face become passive.

Breathing is lower down in the body. There is more diaphragm awareness and abdominal movement.

When humans and animals are deeply relaxed, **Throat Breathing (Ujjayi)** occurs naturally. It is not unusual to hear a human or dog breathing through a slightly closed throat while sleeping or dozing.

1. *It is possible to control the heart beat and other bodily functions but it takes practise and concentration. Some yogis and military personnel, for example, have trained themselves to do this (see* The Psychic Warrior, *by David Morehouse, ISBN 978-190-2636207).*
2. *All creatures with a backbone, e.g. humans, animals and fish, have this basic mechanism.*
3. *Swami Ambikananda, from Reading, UK, said in a workshop that she had asked a cancer specialist why so many people had cancer today. He said,* Because there is too much use of the Sympathetic Nervous System.
4. The Daily Mail, *30.1.08.*

The Brain Page

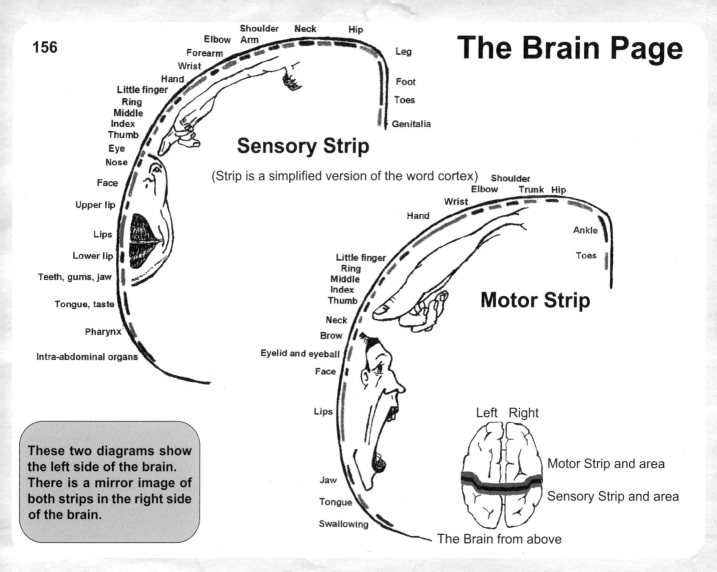

Sensory Strip

(Strip is a simplified version of the word cortex)

Shoulder Neck Hip
Elbow Arm
Forearm
Wrist
Hand
Little finger
Ring
Middle
Index
Thumb
Eye
Nose
Face
Upper lip
Lips
Lower lip
Teeth, gums, jaw
Tongue, taste
Pharynx
Intra-abdominal organs

Leg
Foot
Toes
Genitalia

Motor Strip

Shoulder
Elbow Trunk Hip
Wrist
Hand
Ankle
Toes

Little finger
Ring
Middle
Index
Thumb
Neck
Brow
Eyelid and eyeball
Face
Lips
Jaw
Tongue
Swallowing

These two diagrams show the left side of the brain. There is a mirror image of both strips in the right side of the brain.

Left   Right

Motor Strip and area
Sensory Strip and area
The Brain from above

Observations

IN **Yoga Nidra** we move our awareness around the body, in a systematic and repetitive way. This takes us on a journey round the sensory/motor strips of the brain. As we connect to different parts of the body, the associated nerve pathways are cleared and relaxation induced.

As you can see from the diagram, the hands and face have a large amount of space allocated to them. This explains why hand **Mudras** (the way we hold our hands in meditation and posture work) are so powerful. Each finger has a significant amount of neural connections. Please note, the **diaphragm** doesn't even get a mention.

When we talk about the left and right side of the brain and map the activities of the brain, we are referring to the way most brains function. It is a generalization. Some people, for example, have their verbal centres on the right side of the brain (*see page 4*).

Since about the 1950s, scientists have started to understand about the **neuroplasticity** of the brain. The brain circuits are not fixed and can be altered by experience and with training. We can consciously alter the neurological wiring of the brain. Yoga offers the experience and training that can rewire the brain in a beneficial, healing way.

When part of the brain is injured, the functions of the damaged part can re-establish themselves in another part of the brain. It is possible, for example, for a child to live a fairly normal life if half the brain is removed. With medical assistance, the parts that were disengaged reappear in the remaining half.

Scientists are surprised that some people can live with hardly any brain at all. I know of two people, who were sufferers of **Hydrocephalus** (the cerebrospinal fluid becomes dammed up inside the skull), who were discovered to have a large sack of water instead of a brain, and virtually no brain at all. One had an IQ of 126 and gained an honours degree in mathematics. The other had an IQ of 75, but was not considered mentally retarded or disabled[1].

Also, another brain has recently been discovered in the abdomen. The same type of neurons found in the head and heart brains are found in the large and small intestine. The gut can send and receive impulses, record experiences and respond to emotion, hence the term **gut feeling**. Mantak Chia says; *Western science has shown that the abdomen also has a brain which is connected to the larger brain in the head. The Tao discovered that it is easier to create and store energy in the abdomen than in the head*[2] .

1. www.perdurabo10.com/id1202.html *and* www.newscientist.com/article/dn12301
2. www.ipn.at/ipn.asp?AQB

PATANJALI[1] SAID; *Yoga is a process of uniting the individual soul with the Universal Soul. Yoga is also that state in which the activities of the mind are restrained.*

Yoga uses many different techniques for inducing **Pratyahara[2]**, stopping the mind from wandering off down leafy lanes, and calming the fluctuations of the mind. Here are some examples from this book:

Direction of Thought
This is divided into two sections:

A. Moving the body in different directions. The Swimming Dragon, Figure of Eight Sequence, and Standing Pratyahara.

B. Internally moving awareness round the body. Om Gum Namaha Meditation, Sweeping, Figure of Eight Breathing and Gold Yoga Nidra.

Counting[3]
Square Breathing and Breaths per Minute.

Listening
The Inner Sound in Sensory Meditation, the use of Mantra[4], Om Gum Namaha Meditation and Hamsa Meditation.

More than one technique can be used at the same time. Some people, who try meditation with only a mantra as a point of concentration, lose their confidence and feel discouraged when daily trivia and chatter keep bubbling to the surface. Some minds have to be trained, in the same way that animals are trained, to calm the fluctuations. When using **Direction of Thought** and **Counting**, the mind is kept on track by the established pattern of direction and sequence of numbers. A combination of techniques suits some people better. Some experimentation is necessary.

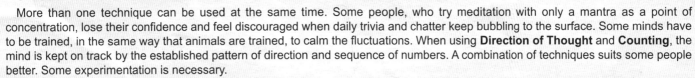

The Brain without Thoughts

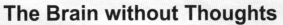

A meditation can still be highly beneficial even when thoughts intrude. Don't be discouraged. Background noise and thoughts are similar in meditation. Some people can meditate in airports and places with unpredictable and inconsistent background noises. Continuous electronic hums and ticking clocks can be more distracting.

The secret is, maybe, not to waste energy on them. Any reaction to them, especially an emotional one, wastes energy. Let them fall on neutral territory, or a blank page. Simply return to your chosen point or points of concentration and direct all your energy through there. It is like directing the warm rays of the sun through a magnifying glass. It generates enough heat to burn objects. Channel your energy the same way during meditation.

The mind calming techniques in this section help us to take our energy way from the verbal centres of the brain, without having to make a conscious effort to do so. There are special times when thoughts almost disappear completely. One occurs when you pause after inhalation and exhalation. These pauses are called **Kumbhaka**. The ancient yogis spent a lot of time practising Kumbhaka. You can experience an empty, hollow space during this time. Another one is when we listen intently. If you ask a group of people to listen to a pin drop, everybody will stop breathing and thinking. Smiling also calms the mind (*see below*).

In his book, *Energy Balancing through the Tao[5]*, Mantak Chia elaborates further. In the chapter entitled *Tan Tien Consciousness: The Second Brain*, he talks about the relationship between the head brain and the abdominal brain. He does not refer to the tiny brain in the heart, and calls the abdominal brain the Second Brain. He says ... *the head brain is a 'monkey mind', riddled with doubt, shame, guilt and suspicion. It is always thinking, planning, worrying ... Scientists have discovered that when people spend a lot of time worrying, their upper (in the head) brain uses a lot of energy. They say the upper brain can use up to 80 per cent of the body's energy, leaving only 20 per cent for the organs.*

We need to use the brain in the head in order to perform complex functions such as reasoning, making plans and making calculations. These are typical left brain functions. However, in our daily life of consciousness, awareness and feeling, which is typically governed by the right brain, we can either use the brain in our head or the brain in the gut.

He goes on to say that you can rest the upper brain by bringing your awareness to the lower brain, which creates and stores energy. You can consciously direct the generated energy from the lower brain to the upper brain and recharge it.

He talks about smiling down into the abdomen. *By just flexing the facial muscles into the position of a genuine smile, we can produce the same effects on the nervous system that naturally go with a natural spontaneous smile. We can actually make ourselves relaxed and happy by taking advantage of this built-in mechanism.... Learning to smile down to the abdominal area ... is the first step in training the second brain ... When the upper brain is resting, brain repair and maintenance occur and new brain cells can grow.* Sometimes we over-work our upper brain and it becomes depleted of energy. Try sending it on a holiday by smiling into the abdomen. Not only is it highly beneficial, it also makes you happy.

Jill Bolte Taylor, PhD., describes in her book, *My Stroke of Insight[6]*, what happened when a stroke in the left side of her brain rendered her verbal centres redundant. She is a brain scientist, artist and musician. She describes, in a charming way, what it is like to live without words. She also adds a spiritual dimension. To find out more, visit YouTube: **How it feels to have a stroke**. To me this is essential information for anybody interested in meditation, the mind and enlightenment. Her contributions are, very wisely, included in the Dru Yoga Teachers Training Course.

1. *Patanjali compiled thousands of years of yogic wisdom in his sutras (threads of thought) sometime between 200 BC and 200 AD. This is the first sutra of Samadhi Pada.*

2. *Please refer to the Glossary.*

3. *Patanjali wrote in Sutra 34, Samadhi Pada:* The mind becomes purified and clear with regular practise of pranayama. *The yogis of old, according to the Hatha Yoga Pradipika, appeared to have spent more time doing alternative nostril breathing than anything else. The recommended practice involved counting in ratios for 40 rounds, four times a day, with breath retentions.*

4. *Please refer to the Glossary.*

5. Energy Balance through the Tao *by Mantak Chia, Destiny Books, 1999. ISBN 1-59477-059-X*

6. My Stroke of Insight *by Jill Bolte Taylor, Ph.D., Viking, 2006. ISBN 978-0-670-02074-4*

Sweeping

SWEEPING IS a technique for observing the sensations throughout the body. It has Buddhist roots, and can be practised lying on your back or sitting.

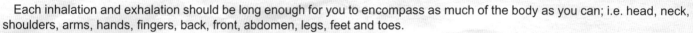

Method

1. Bring your awareness to the top of your head. **INHALE** with full attention.
2. **EXHALE** slowly, sweeping your awareness through your body from head to feet.
3. **INHALE.** Let your awareness creep up the body from feet to head.

Each inhalation and exhalation should be long enough for you to encompass as much of the body as you can; i.e. head, neck, shoulders, arms, hands, fingers, back, front, abdomen, legs, feet and toes.

After reading an article by Deepak Chopra on *Quantum Physics and Consciousness*, I broadened out this practice[1]. I started to 'sweep', concentrating on different aspects of our being. This developed into **The Five Aspects**. I usually do each aspect for three breaths. You may choose to do more.

The Five Aspects

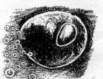

1. Body as heavy, solid matter.
2. Body as liquid.
3. Body as vibrating energy.
4. Body as empty space.
5. Body connecting to the waves of energy that underlie all matter.

Empty space in cells

Electric neurons (above), and a healthy cell being attacked by viral intruders (left).

1. Body as heavy matter. This is the way we think about our bodies in everyday life. We perceive solid bone and muscle. A relaxed person is very heavy, as anybody will discover if they try to lift a completely drunk person. Allow yourself to feel very heavy.

2. Body as liquid. Between 70 and 80 per cent of our body is liquid. The blood transports oxygen all over the body. There are the equivalent of estuaries, rivers, tributaries and little streams all over the body.

3. Body as vibrating energy.

Deepak Chopra says *... **The human body is made up of atoms. The atoms in turn are made up of subatomic particles that are moving at lightning speeds around huge empty space. And the subatomic particles are not material things. They are fluctuations of energy and information in a void.... Einstein clearly showed that energy and matter were essentially the same thing. One only needs to add one more ingredient: information.*** Everything in the universe is vibration at its own frequency, whether it is a slab of concrete, a leaf, a note from a musical instrument or an emotion.

4. Body as empty space.

Experienced through the senses, the body appears to have substance but the senses are unreliable. Seen through the eyes of a physicist, the body is 99.9999 per cent empty space. The English physicist, Sir Arthur Eddington (1882-1944), said that if you took away the empty space from all the six billion people that were then on the planet, you could compress all the subatomic particles into a volume only a little larger than a grain of rice.

5. Body experienced as the waves of energy that underlie all matter.

Ultimately that 0.0001 per cent that appears to be matter is also empty space. Wayne Dyer says *... **you find atoms, then electrons, then subatomic particles, until you finally go as small as is possible, with a microscope at full magnification. Here you will find there are no particles, but waves of energy that mysteriously come and go** [2]*.

Try to scan up and down the body and imagine these mysterious waves of energy. Ultimately the waves and energy are the same thing. This is the essence of **Yoga Vedanta** philosophy. The missing ingredient is the information that changes the waves into the particles that make up your body.

1. *Living Yoga (interview with S.N. Goenka), Tarcher/Putnam. ISBN 0-87477-729-1*
2. *Manifest your Destiny by Dr Wayne Dyer, Element, 2003. ISBN 0-00-717046-1*

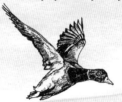

Hamsa Meditation

This meditation involves **mantra** and **visualization**. **Hamsa** means **flying swan** or **goose** in Sanskrit. **INHALE** as you think **Ham** and **EXHALE** as you think **Sa**.

It uses the right side of the brain where long term visual memory is stored in the Hippocampus. You are going to imagine you are a flying bird in familiar territory. You will be creating pictures of places you remember. The mantra is a stabilizing ingredient that floats in the background. If you find it difficult to visualize and mentally repeat the mantra, just bring it back into your mind when thoughts intrude.

Memory is much more acute when you are relaxed. Take advantage of the relaxed state your posture work will have induced.

Variations on this theme

1. At the end of a yoga class, I sometimes talk my pupils through a journey, from where we are to a place they all know. Then I give them about five minutes to fly back by themselves, taking a different route. We only use the mantra when I'm not talking.
2. You can visit your favourite place and fly around all the little nooks and crannies and dark mysterious places you love so much. You may be surprised at all the detail you can remember.
3. Leonardo Da Vinci, 1452-1519, the Italian multi-talented genius, used to hate seeing birds locked up in cages. He used to buy the birds and then let them go. Imagine you are one of his birds and he takes you to the countryside and lets you go. Fly around for the first time.

THIS BEAUTIFUL meditation was given to me by Swami Isa of Trivandrum in Kerala, India. I visited him while staying at the Sivananda Ashram, Neyyar Dam in 2001. With his permission, I taught it every week for five years during my meditation classes at Inglewood Health Hydro.

Om Gum Namaha is the mantra of Ganesh, the elephant-like aspect of God, the remover of obstacles and boundaries. When an elephant comes towards you, you get out of the way. I think of this meditation as mind-expanding and obstacle-removing.

Method

1. Sing the mantra out loud a few times on the same note, and then internalize the vibrations (think it). In this meditation there are two breaths per repetition of each mantra.

2. Sit in a comfortable meditation posture. Let the hands rest in **Chin Mudra** (thumb and first finger together), or another simple hand mudra, on the tops of the thighs.

3. Bring your awareness to the base of the spine. **INHALE** and think **Om**, as you trace your awareness from the base of the spine to the top of the spine. If you have difficulty doing this, visualize a white or silver light moving up the spine.

4. EXHALE as you think **Gum** and bring your awareness from the top of the spine to the top of your forehead.

5. INHALE and think **Namaha** as you bring your awareness to the top of your head. Let it hover a short distance above your head.

6. Your second exhalation is long and silent. Imagine your aura and energy floating down from the top of your head, outside the body, in an oval shape, to the base of the spine.
Repeat the cycle as many times as you want to.

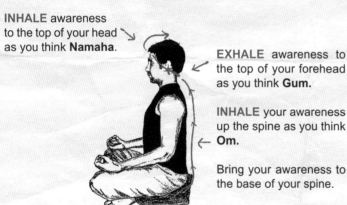

INHALE awareness to the top of your head as you think **Namaha**.

EXHALE awareness to the top of your forehead as you think **Gum**.

INHALE your awareness up the spine as you think **Om**.

Bring your awareness to the base of your spine.

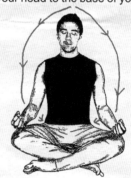

EXHALE your aura and energy from the top of your head to the base of your spine.

Observations

During the long silent exhalation, as your awareness floats from the top of the head to the base of the spine, people experience different things. Some see sparkling lights, like sparkler fireworks. A few people in the class said they saw somebody standing in front of them. You may see different colours. Just let your mind drift, without expectation, and observe what happens.

This meditation seemed to suit a lot of people. One lady in the class said it would be good on tube trains (the underground). I tried it out the next time I went to London and discovered that it was.

Comments from Swami Isa

Swami Isa calls this meditation ***basic energy tuning***. I wrote to him to get his permission to use it in my books. He did say I could use it, but he had reservations. I received this reply from his ashram:

Actually printing a mantra is not very useful, because 'the real power in a mantra is given directly from the Guru or Master in the mantra initiation'. Swami said; 'Only someone who has been initiated by a Master can properly chant that mantra and receive its benefits.' He asked that if you print it, you advise your readers it is not intended for their own practice. If you want to practise a mantra, you should seek out a Guru or Master for initiation.

Swami said; 'In the mantra initiation process, it is an exchange of vital energy or a prana-to-prana exchange.' That is not possible from printed or other media, because 'mantras are pranic, not printed material.'

Further, when Swami initiates someone directly into a mantra, He has the opportunity to make adjustments to 'how much force, vibration or feeling that individual needs to apply,' and to coach them accordingly. That is why a personal interaction is also very necessary.

To create interest, OK! But don't miss the importance of a real Guru.

This is the traditional approach to mantra meditation. In the light of this tradition, printing it here is a compromise, but some compromises still have much to offer. My pupils have benefited from practising it and I hope you do too.

For more information about Swami Isa, please visit www.isalayan.com

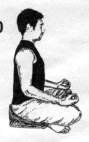

Sensory Meditation

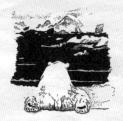

THIS IS a meditation I have developed myself. It is my particular way of entering the meditative state. Occasionally I teach it at the end of my lessons, either in a sitting position or lying on our backs. As some people have found it helpful, I am sharing it with you here.

Try to become familiar with your **Inner Sound** before you start this meditation. There are many different internal sounds that are heard on the journey of spiritual development. The particular sound I concentrate on is the high pitched electronic vibration you might hear late at night, when it is dark and quiet and you put your head on the pillow before going to sleep.

Some people never hear it, but others can train themselves to pick it up whenever they want. I became interested in it when I heard that some Buddhist monks used it during meditation.

I was directed to a website in 2001 (*www.ipn.at/ipn.asp?BJE*). The **Bio Feedback Institute** in Vienna explained it and I have used it ever since. To hear the **Inner Sound** please visit my website, www.koolkatpublications.co.uk

Method

1. Become aware of the movement of the diaphragm and the completely relaxed abdomen. Slow down your breathing, especially your exhalations. Prepare to take a journey inwards.

2. Choose a simple mantra (see Glossary) of one or two syllables. **Om (Aum)**, **Sham** (pronounced Sharm, this is another name for Lord Krishna), **So Hum** and **Sat Nam** are the ones that come to mind.

3. Start off with the hands in **Chin Mudra** (thumbs and first fingers together) and your eyes closed.

4. Internalize your mantra. The first breath when you meditate is important. Give it your full attention. If your mantra has one syllable, think it each time you inhale and each time you exhale. If it has two syllables think the first one on the inhalation and the second on the exhalation.

5. Continue breathing and repeating your mantra until you feel the breath becoming calm and peaceful and the pauses between inhalation and exhalation becoming longer.

6. When you feel ready, add more points of concentration. First, look at the colours you see when your eyes are closed. Observe the movement of the colours. Some people only see black when their eyes are closed. Just do the best you can.

7. Now try to hear your **inner sound**. It may help if you tilt your head slightly forwards and concentrate on the top of your forehead.

8. Continue with your breath, mantra, inner vision and inner sound for as long as you feel you need to.

9. When you feel the time is right, open out your hands, with the palms facing upwards. Bring your awareness to your left hand thumb. Connect to one finger per breath, i.e. per inhalation and exhalation, and then move on to the next finger. After 10 breaths you will have reached the right hand thumb. Repeat the breath on the right hand thumb and then work your way back for another 10 breaths to the left hand thumb.

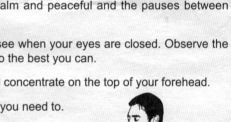

Just carry on for as long as you want to. You are now internalizing your sense of touch. Bring your awareness to your finger tips. You may want to move each finger a little as you connect to it.

10. Try to go for a certain number of fingers without a single thought coming into your mind. Some people have no difficulty going for five fingers without any thoughts intruding, others find it very difficult. It does improve with practice. If you find it difficult, try going for two or three breaths and slowly build up. Once you have had a thoughtless mind for about eight breaths it is easier to go for much longer. Listening to the **inner sound** helps.

11. When the ripples of your mind are sufficiently still and calm, take your awareness to the **Heart Centre** (see page 4). Let the breath become soft and gentle ... Breathe into it emotional warmth and light. Gently smile down into the **Heart Centre**.

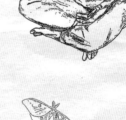

You may observe a change in your breathing. It may slow down and almost disappear. Your connection to the diaphragm may feel more subtle and have a different quality. With the change in breathing there comes a deep peace. Perhaps this is where the practice changes from concentration to meditation.

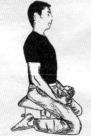
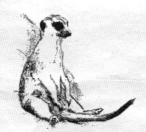
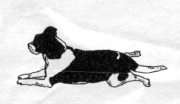
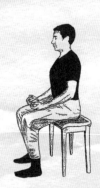

also from YogaWords

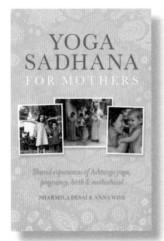

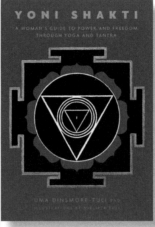

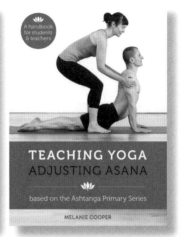

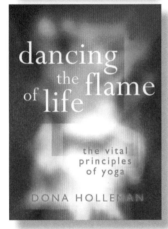

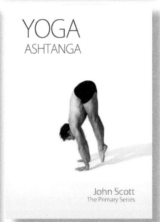

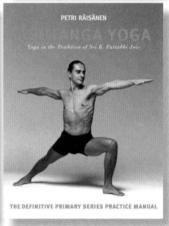

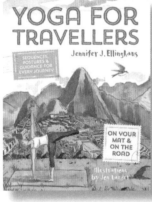

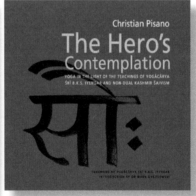

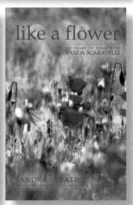

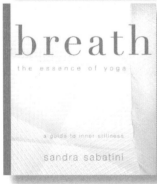

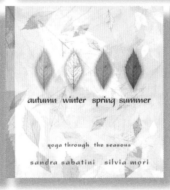

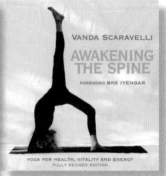

www.pinterandmartin.com